Viral Sex

Viral Sex

The Nature of AIDS

Jaap Goudsmit

Oxford University Press
New York   *Oxford*

Oxford University Press

Oxford   New York
Athens   Auckland   Bangkok   Bogotá   Bombay
Buenos Aires   Calcutta   Cape Town   Dar es Salaam
Delhi   Florence   Hong Kong   Istanbul   Karachi
Kuala Lumpur   Madras   Madrid   Melbourne
Mexico City   Nairobi   Paris   Singapore
Taipei   Tokyo   Toronto

and associated companies in
Berlin   Ibadan

Library of Congress Cataloging-in-Publication Data
Goudsmit, Jaap, 1951–
Viral sex : the nature of AIDS / by Jaap Goudsmit.
p. cm.   Includes bibliographical references and index.
ISBN 0-19-509728-9
1. HIV (Viruses)   2. HIV infections.   I. Title.
QR414.6.H58G68   1997
614.5'993—dc20   96-27910

ISBN 0-19-512496-0 (Pbk.)
9 8 7 6 5 4 3 2 1

Dedicated to
Tine van der Waals–Koenigs (1915–1995)

Contents

Acknowledgments

After more than ten years of AIDS research, I felt the need to share with a wider audience what I have learned from the work of my group and other scientists in the field of retrovirology. The result is this book, which could not have appeared without the help and stimulation of many people, both scientists and nonscientists. My own work has been inspired by many scientists I have met and worked with, but two in particular.

One of these mentors was D. Carleton Gajdusek, who showed me the importance of constantly crossing the boundaries between basic and applied science and between the social and the biomedical sciences. He taught me never to forget, as I attempt to unravel the pathology and epidemiology of a disease, the patient who suffers with the disease.

The other source of inspiration was Manfred Eigen, who introduced me to the evolutionary aspects of retrovirus behavior. He led me to think about retrovirus evolution in terms of populations or, in his term, "quasi-species." My work has been greatly influenced by his concept of RNA sequence space. This envisions a viral universe in which RNA virus and retrovirus populations with related but nonidentical sets of genetic information follow their trajectory not as individual viruses but as swarms with one master sequence as the center of gravity.

Once I had written the book, three individuals above all brought it to its final form. First, Lucy Phillips acted as my personal editor. She also provided indispensable advice on the presentation of my ideas to a nonspecialist audience. If the book gives pleasure, you as the reader and I as the writer owe this to her ingenuity and her enormous commitment over the last two years. Second and third, Song Ding edited the visuals, assisted by Wim van Est. The illustrations appear as they do because of their continuous support and meticulous care. These three people could not have made a better team for me. I can only hope that they enjoyed our work together as much as I did.

I began writing the book in 1993 during a sabbatical year spent largely at the Aaron Diamond AIDS Research Center in New York City. The support I felt in that environment has shaped the book in a major way. The center's director, David Ho, read each chapter and, without making him responsible for anything I wrote, I must thank him for his immense influence on my thinking. Without his continuous feedback and encouragement I could never have completed this project.

I must also thank Irene Diamond, a nonscientist with great appreciation for science. She has almost single-handedly shaped AIDS research in the New York area through her support of the Aaron Diamond Foundation. My conversations with her gave me all the reasons I needed to tackle this book. Her dedication to AIDS research in all its complexities, from the ethical and social issues to the basic science of HIV and antiviral progress, is an overwhelming and inspiring example for all who know her.

Most of my writing was done at Point Lookout, New York. This Long Island haven with its Dutch landscape provided optimal conditions for the work. I was grateful not only for the view of the ocean but even more for the company of the Binkhorst family. Sonja Binkhorst, with her daughter, Audrey, and sons, Mark and Gordon, were mirror and sounding board to every idea as it matured to a full concept. These four friends also gave me and my family a strong feeling of home in the United States.

In particular, Audrey and Mark made a unique contribution. Their faith in my enterprise was so strong that late one night they searched the trash cans in a New York neighborhood where part of my manuscript had disappeared from Mark's car. And because of their devotion to the cause, a miracle occurred: most of the stolen pages were recovered from the garbage on the streets of Manhattan.

Of course, to write a book is impossible without those people who fill in for you and put up with your distracted state. I am indebted to my colleagues at the Academic Medical Center in Amsterdam. In our new Department of Human Retrovirology (formerly the Human Retrovirus Laboratory), I must especially thank the doctoral and postdoctoral students and the laboratory technicians who encountered, on too many occasions, an absentminded chief preoccupied by monkeys. As an excuse I will say that the book became part of many other projects, and many projects became part of the book. In this lucky process of cross-fertilization, two individuals deserve special mention. The first is Frank de Wolf, associate professor in our department, who stood in for me many times in some very difficult situations. The other is Niek Urbanus, dean of the medical faculty and chairman of the Medical Center board, who allowed me the 1993 sabbatical and, on my return, created the new retrovirus department.

A book is also impossible without someone like Kirk Jensen, senior editor at Oxford University Press, who guided the project throughout and kept faith until its conclusion.

Above all, I owe everything to my wife, Fransje, and my daughters, Judith, Leah, and Keziah. Only because of their patience, which at times I did not deserve, was I able to reach the end of this book. Just after Fransje successfully defended her Ph.D. thesis, she graciously sent me off to Rome for World AIDS Day, December 1, 1995. There I wrote the last chapter and the epilogue, concluding this marathon of more than two years. I am very lucky to have such a family and can now enjoy spending more time with them.

Rome
December 4, 1995

Introduction

I t now seems incredible that AIDS went largely unnoticed and un-
named until the early 1980s. Suddenly an escalating number of cases
were reported from the United States, Europe, and Africa, indicating
the onset of a worldwide siege. The disease is now rampant, particularly in
Africa, where it is killing men and women of reproductive age as well as
children infected at birth. It is rapidly moving into Asia and South America.
In these areas, as in Africa, it is usually transmitted by heterosexual relations, perinatal infection, and contaminated blood supplies or hospital
equipment. Meanwhile, AIDS is changing character in the United States
and Europe. At first spread largely by homosexual relations and intravenous
drug use, it is now infecting more women and children, mainly those of the
inner city.

The AIDS threat has mobilized an unprecedented research effort to understand and control the disease. We have discovered its agent, the human
immunodeficiency virus (HIV). Every day we know more about this complex
retrovirus and how it works, but still we lack an effective defense strategy.

HIV is not new to the world or to the primate family, which includes
monkeys, apes, and humans. It is descended from a virus that in various

guises has long infected, or colonized, certain African apes and monkeys. Analogous to HIV, it has been named simian immunodeficiency virus (SIV), although it causes no immunodeficiency or disease in these natural hosts. It is harmless to them but lethal to naive, or unaccustomed, primate hosts such as humans.

The question is why, after millennia of contact between African monkeys and humans, has SIV only now entered the human population as HIV? Why is this virus so lethal, and what can we do about it?

As this book explains, the answers must be found in the virus itself. We must realize that like any virus—indeed, like any organism—HIV seeks only to survive. It has no evil intent but simply needs a host in which it can reproduce. Its offspring need a new host where they can repeat the cycle, and so on. Retroviruses inhabit many nonhuman species without causing disease. Each has slowly adapted to its particular species and prefers to spread among those familiar hosts. But by accident or necessity, a virus sometimes jumps to a new species. For HIV, we are a relatively new host, a new environment with problems.

The main problem is, this virus that we fear so much is not actually very contagious or infectious. When you stick yourself with a nonsterile needle, you are far more likely to get a hepatitis virus than the AIDS virus. So HIV has tried to evolve toward higher efficiency of transmission among humans. To do this, it has increased its rate of reproduction to achieve and sustain a high level of circulating virus in our bodily fluids, especially blood and semen. Since HIV happens to reproduce primarily in crucial cells of our immune system, its high level of production eventually causes immunodeficiency, AIDS, and death.

A first step against HIV is to lower the persistently high virus load that destroys the human immune system. If we can keep it low, the virus may change genes to survive. It may find ways to spread effectively without causing disease. Then we would have the kind of equilibrium or mutual accommodation that we see with monkeys and their SIV.

Unfortunately, HIV is just as likely to find ways to spread that cause disease *despite* low virus load. HIV does not seek to harm, but it does not seek *not* to harm. A virus does not know or care. So our next step is to take genetic control of HIV and disconnect its need to spread from its disease-causing effects. We must reengineer its evolutionary pathway so it can survive and spread without causing AIDS. The reengineered HIV, or key parts of it, could then be introduced into the at-risk community for protection against more dangerous members of the HIV family.

To engineer such a change is not impossible or even far-fetched. The technology is within reach if we sufficiently understand the nature of HIV: its evolution, family tree, and peculiar habits. This book takes the reader on a personal exploration of this retrovirus. It looks at HIV from new angles and tells where we might go from here.

The Retrovirus and Its Key Enzyme

But what is a retrovirus, and what makes it such a formidable opponent? These unique viruses were characterized and named by the late Howard Temin, who, with David Baltimore, received the Nobel Prize in 1975. Temin and Baltimore, working independently, discovered reverse transcriptase, the wonder enzyme that allows retroviruses to do what, until 1970, was considered impossible: convert RNA to DNA. The central dogma of biology was just the opposite: DNA produces RNA, which then produces proteins. Temin spent his life studying retroviruses, which were found to cause cancer in many species, including humans. They were also found to cause AIDS, the most frightening infection we have ever encountered.

In all retroviruses, the genetic material consists of genes strung along two single strands of RNA. This material, the genome, is packaged in a protein envelope. Once the virus has infected a particular cell, reverse transcriptase goes into action. It converts the two RNA strands into DNA, which is spliced into the DNA of the host cell. Buried in the host genome and the genetic code, the virus can sooner or later add its own subversive instructions to those of the host genes. From then on, the host cell machinery cannot escape helping the retrovirus to reproduce. However, the viral imposter is often dormant until triggered by particular conditions. Since HIV infects immune cells, it is triggered to reproduce when they are activated by some foreign invader. As they multiply to fight the invader, HIV multiplies too.

Retroviruses infect various types of cells in various species. Some can infect several types of cells. Some, like HIV, can infect only a limited number. The infection may or may not cause disease. It may last only the lifetime of a single host or be passed down for generations. Some retroviruses have inhabited various mammal species for thousands of years and are now permanently part of the species genome.

When retroviruses finally reproduce, they make up for lost time. They continually generate an unusually large population of infectious particles, or virions. Each day the host is infected with what Temin called a "viral swarm" of about a billion virions. It includes an unusual range of strain variants, or hybrids. Manfred Eigen, another Nobelist (who showed that life on earth most likely began with RNA), called such a virus population a "quasi-species." Its size and diversity give the retrovirus flexibility and resilience. Many variants are nonviable (i.e., they cannot reproduce), and many viable variants succumb to the host defense system. But out of the huge swarm, many survivors remain. The virus appears to rely on the best variants while sacrificing those that are weak or deleterious. Of course, the virus actually does nothing. It has no brain or plan. The selection process is random and ongoing. The fittest variants survive as long as they are the fittest, then others take their place.

Retrovirus adaptation to new environments results in part from sloppy cloning. This produces inexact copies that occasionally, by sheer chance, improve on the original. But adaptation results mainly from what Temin called "retroviral sex." This drives the evolution of viruses like HIV by salvaging the most functional and fit variants. In fact, viral sex is central to the very nature of HIV and AIDS.

Viral Sex and Recombination

As humans, we tend to think that reproduction is always sexual. However, strictly speaking, sex means the mating of two parents and the reassortment or recombination of two distinct sets of genes. Most often, viruses and other microorganisms reproduce by asexual methods. Each organism replicates its own genetic material so, barring error, asexual offspring are clones or exact copies of a single parent. In sexual reproduction, offspring are a new creation, a blend of two parental sets of genes. Sexual offspring are exact copies only under conditions avoided by most humans: the mating of identical twins.

Retroviruses can clone or copy themselves, but they can also reproduce sexually. Other viruses can too, but retroviruses are more sexually adept and active, and they gain more benefits. Most higher animals procreate mainly at specific fertile times. Retroviruses procreate at any time. This may sound like humans, but while humans can mate at any time, they are fertile only at intervals. Their mating does not always produce offspring. The mating of retroviruses always does, and they number not one or two but millions.

Retroviruses are like other mating organisms in that offspring are generally more or less like the parents. However, under certain circumstances viral sex can produce recombinants that show major change—far more change than would ever be seen in normal human offspring.

Sex for retroviruses is a two-stage process (see Figure I.1). The first begins when two retroviruses infect the same cell. If identical, each having the same two strands of RNA, they will produce offspring that show little or no change. But if each has a distinct set of RNA, the parents will produce offspring of three kinds. Two will be homozygous, having either two identical strands of RNA from one parent or two identical strands from the other parent. The third will be heterozygous, having two different RNA strands, one from each parent.

The second stage begins when a cell is infected by heterozygous virions. When they mate, reverse transcriptase shuffles the RNA strands while converting them to DNA, producing recombinants of the two parents. Most of these offspring are not markedly different from the parents; a few are deleterious and die. But sometimes a recombinant has spectacular new features. If these features make the virus more suitable for survival in the hostile world of the host, with its tendency to eliminate the virus by immunity, this newborn virus will quickly outcompete less suitable strains. It may conquer the world.

Recombination allows retroviruses to maintain a pool of variants with differential ability to spread under changing environmental circumstances. One never knows what they will do next. They are prepared to adapt to almost any change, including a change of hosts or route of transmission. As this book will tell, HIV has already adapted to a human host. Spread mainly through sexual intercourse, HIV found ample opportunity to spread to epidemic proportions when it encountered highly promiscuous subgroups of homosexuals in Europe and heterosexuals in Africa and South America. Some HIVs became efficient at anal transmission, while others became efficient at vaginal transmission. All the while, the virus was increasing its production to spread better, which incidentally caused AIDS.

But AIDS is only the latest chapter in the history of HIV. Tracing that history, this book will show that the AIDS virus is far older than the AIDS

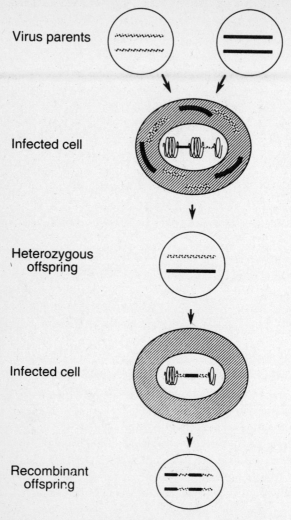

Virus parents

Infected cell

Heterozygous offspring

Infected cell

Recombinant offspring

Figure I.1 **Viral sex and recombination as seen with retroviruses.** *Production of viruses with new properties requires nonidentical but compatible parent viruses, i.e., parents with distinct RNA genomes but enough overlap to permit genetic crossover (a). When they infect a cell, their RNA is converted to DNA and spliced into the cell genome (b). Particles of the integrated viruses mate and produce heterozygotes, i.e., offspring whose RNA includes a strand from each parent (c). When heterozygotes infect a cell and enter the genome (d), they produce recombinants, i.e., offspring with two identical RNA strands, each a mosaic of genes and gene fragments from both parents (e). (Coffin 1993; Temin 1991.)*

epidemic. This virus needed millennia of evolution and many changes of host to emerge. Even then, it could not cause AIDS until it began to circulate rapidly among us. AIDS is a uniquely human disease because it could only develop with rapid human sexual transmission.

Viral sex gives HIV an important edge, but it also gives us a weapon. The key to the AIDS problem lies, in part, in human sexual behavior but also, ironically, in the sexual behavior of HIV. We may find viral nature easier to change than human nature. But even if we can manipulate the procreation of HIV to control AIDS, we must be forewarned. Monkeys and other animals peacefully harbor many microbes whose potential is as threatening to humans as HIV. The animals and their microbes are content in their equilibrium, but if we destroy the animals or their habitat, the microbes will need a new host. Like HIV, microbes that find a foothold in a human host could use viral sex to adapt, with human disease as a consequence.

Viral Sex

1

The Most Disarming Virus

In the early 1980s, a strange new epidemic emerged among North American homosexual men. It was first seen in the large gay communities of New York and California among young men who were very sexually active. These men became mysteriously ill with infections and tumors that, according to previous experience, were rarely serious and rarely combined in the same individual. Certainly they had never been seen in epidemic proportions in such a narrowly defined risk group.

One of the infectious agents was *Pneumocystis carinii*, a usually harmless microorganism that thrives around us and even inside of us. Like many other organisms in our environment, *P. carinii* routinely colonizes most of us, at an early age, with no ill effects under ordinary circumstances. Colonization of one organism by another—also called *infection*—quite often causes no disease. Although *P. carinii* had been known to cause serious and sometimes fatal pneumonia in humans and other animals, this happened only in circumstances of abnormal weakness. It might harm malnourished children or severely ill people with a lowered capability to fight infections, but not vigorous young men.

The same was generally true for Kaposi's sarcoma (KS), the tumor most often seen in the new epidemic. This cancer is recognized by bluish red skin lesions that usually appear first on the feet and lower legs. The lesions tend to spread upward on the body, and may also spread inward from the skin, especially to the lymph nodes. KS had previously been seen in aging men in the United States and Europe, but it was uncommon and rarely aggressive. It was more frequent and serious in Africa, but still no great threat.

What was going on among these young gay men? Physicians who treated them in San Francisco, Los Angeles, and New York soon found that they suffered massive immunodeficiency. Some impairment of the immune system that normally protects us from invaders had allowed the bizarre and fatal combination of infections and tumors. The condition was marked by a rapid decline of certain blood cells, or T-helper cells, whose cell wall includes a crucial molecule known as CD4.

These CD4-positive cells are major players in our immune system. CD4+ cells are essential to fight all types of invaders. In this epidemic, their impairment was apparently not inborn but somehow acquired, so the disorder came to be called AIDS: acquired immunodeficiency syndrome.

How had these young homosexual men acquired such a severe immune disturbance? Clues began to come from the US Centers for Disease Control (CDC) in Atlanta, Georgia. The CDC found that those who developed AIDS had invariably had sex with someone who concurrently had AIDS or later developed the disease. Apparently it was transmitted sexually, most likely by means of seminal fluid.

Then AIDS began to occur among hemophiliacs, but not by sexual transmission. Hemophilia is a congenital disease, seen only in men, in which the blood does not clot normally. It is effectively treated with transfusions of blood that contains clotting factors, but apparently blood could also transmit AIDS. This transmission route was later confirmed when AIDS appeared among intravenous drug users who had shared needles with infected gay men. Intravenous (IV) drug use and needle sharing are not uncommon among the most sexually active gay men, who often combine certain drugs with sexual relations.

The transmission of AIDS in semen and blood, its epidemic spread, and its sudden occurrence in otherwise healthy men suggested an infectious agent, probably a virus. In 1982 or 1983, only two years into the epidemic, a likely suspect was found at the Institut Pasteur of Paris by Françoise Barré-Sinoussi, Jean-Claude Chermann, Luc Montagnier, and colleagues.

The new virus was discovered in an enlarged lymph node taken from a young homosexual man. He had not yet developed AIDS, but AIDS patients were found to have the same virus in their blood.

In 1984, American researchers Mika Popovic, Bob Gallo, and colleagues showed that most AIDS patients had this virus, while a control group of healthy subjects did not. (With today's finer techniques, they would have found the virus in all their AIDS patients.) Meanwhile, the virus infected three lab workers who later developed AIDS. As far as most scientists were concerned, this tragedy supplied the last piece of the puzzle. According to a reasoning process based on Koch's postulates, an agent is linked to a disease in four steps. First, the agent is observed in every case of the disease. Second, it is isolated from people with the disease, then grown in pure culture. Third, the culture causes the disease when inoculated into susceptible subjects (in this case, the unfortunate lab workers). Fourth, the agent is observed and recovered from the experimentally infected subjects.

Some problems would later arise from this early work of the French and American groups, as discussed in Chapter 2. But these researchers identified the new virus, and the Gallo team grew the virus to high levels of infectivity, enabling rapid production of kits to diagnose the infection. The virus was soon known as HIV: human immunodeficiency virus. Perhaps no other virus in history has become so widely known in so short a time.

But what exactly is a virus? Why is HIV so especially deadly? Viruses are infectious agents like bacteria, but they are far smaller and unlike bacteria, not self-sufficient. They are parasites that need a host, like mistletoe needs the oak tree. They can often exist on their own, in a kind of suspended animation, but to reproduce they must use and subvert the mechanisms of a host cell. Some viruses can thrive in only one type of cell within one type of plant or animal. Others are not so fussy. HIV prefers certain T-helper cells and macrophages of the human immune system. (*Macrophage* means "big eater" in Greek because these defender cells neutralize invaders by engulfing and digesting them.) HIV enters its chosen cells through the CD4 molecule mentioned earlier. This crucial discovery was made simultaneously by two groups: David Klatzmann, Jean-Claude Gluckmann, and collaborators in Paris, and Gus Dalgleish, Robin Weiss, and coworkers in London.

Of course, CD4 does not exist solely to give passage to HIV. It did not evolve to serve as the HIV receptor or welcome mat. In fact, its main job is sentry duty: it recognizes intruders and arouses various fighter cells against them. In an ironic twist, HIV uses this guardian molecule to enter and ultimately destroy the cells that carry it on their surface. To ensure its own survival, HIV defends by attacking: it cripples the immune system that would destroy or control it. Its effects are slow to show because, up to a point, the cells it destroys can be replenished. But eventually its steady killing reduces the quantity and quality of CD4+ cells, causing immunodeficiency. By the time people have full-blown AIDS, they cannot cope with invading organisms that normal people accommodate or fight off every day.

The organisms that threaten AIDS patients are not only invaders from our external environment but insiders like *P. carinii*. These members of our internal ecosystem—our natural flora—are usually kept in their place by many factors, including a healthy immune system. But given the opportunity to overgrow or grow in the wrong place, they can cause "opportunistic" infection. Several studies of the natural course of AIDS have shown that certain opportunistic infections always become fatal once HIV is acquired and persists in the blood and other organs of the body.

Where did this treacherous and apparently new virus come from? As the Bible says, "There is no new thing under the sun." HIV may be truly new, but it is more likely an old virus that has gained a new level of virulence, enabling it to cause human immunodeficiency. Or perhaps it has always been virulent but has only now entered the human species.

If so, what animals previously harbored this virus, and where on earth? Why have we not seen AIDS-like disease in these animals? Is AIDS unique to humans? Has the disease appeared before, sporadic and unrecognized, or is it entirely new to this century? If sporadic in the past, why is it suddenly a raging epidemic?

Many questions occur, but the quintessential ones are: Why us and why now?

When AIDS was first seen in North America and then in Europe and Africa, epidemiologists were baffled. Most epidemics can be traced to one focal point, but this one seemed to be spreading independently on three continents. North American and European AIDS were soon regarded as one epidemic, brought to Europe from America by gay men. (As noted in Chapter 2, evidence now shows it traveled the opposite way.) Meanwhile, a different type of AIDS surfaced among a few central Africans living in Belgium and France. This disease was transmitted heterosexually, appeared mainly in women, and had come directly from Africa.

Today AIDS is generally accepted to be more than one epidemic caused by a whole family of HIV types, subtypes, and strains. The main epidemic in North America and Europe is caused by HIV type 1 (HIV-1). Now spreading fast to South America, this Western HIV is apparently becoming ever more lethal or virulent as it is passaged through the human population. That is, it gains strength each time it enters a new person, reproduces in the CD4+ cells, then bursts out to circulate and infect another person.

Unfortunately for us, this process of cycling to virulence seems to be an HIV family trait. (Both *virus* and *virulence* stem from Latin *virus*, meaning "poison" or "venom.") All members of the family, including HIV-1, were probably much less deadly when they first encountered humans. They had to reach a threshold of cycles and new infections before they could cause AIDS and premature death. If so, then HIV may have been with us for millennia. It can suddenly cause AIDS because of some change in us or in its own makeup. For example, HIV may only recently have acquired the mutations or genes to cause human immunodeficiency.

If HIV virulence rises with new infections, are there some types among us that do not yet cause AIDS? So far, research indicates that all members of the HIV family can cause AIDS (some faster than others)—but a very few people can block the disease. We have seen two of these lucky individuals in an Amsterdam study of men infected since 1983. Our study began with a sample of more than one thousand gay men, who were examined every three months. These subjects belonged to the subgroup known to be at highest risk for AIDS: young gay men who seek rough and anonymous sex with multiple partners. Some of the sample were HIV-infected before the study began, but we focused on those who became infected as the study proceeded. These men, who so far number about fifty, have now been followed for an average of ten to twelve years.

As usual with HIV-1, each case started with acute infection. Though brief and sometimes hardly noticeable, this flulike illness was accompanied by the generation of permanent and specific HIV antibodies. Our immune system normally greets any invader by producing specific antibodies. They remain forever on call, should the invader reappear. If it does, they are geared to recognize and tag it as an enemy to be destroyed. HIV antibodies are evidence of seropositivity. Their appearance signifies seroconversion: the first point at which serum is found to contain the virus, its genetic material, or antibodies to the virus. (Tests that show a person to be HIV-positive usually detect antibodies. They are indirect but long-lasting evidence of the virus. Their persistence tends to make them more reliable as evidence than the virus itself or its genetic material.) The acute stage was followed by a period free of symptoms or disease, which usually lasted several years. But of those infected early in the study, more than 75 percent have now developed AIDS, and twenty-three have died. Three individuals developed the disease within only eighteen months of initial infection. At the opposite end of the spectrum, the two lucky ones still show no sign of immunodeficiency.

Incidentally, our work offers further proof that HIV is the agent of AIDS. Of the twenty-three men who died, each acquired HIV infection before development of any immune disturbance. And not a single case of AIDS—or any sign of immunodeficiency—has developed among the many hundreds of men who have remained HIV-negative over the years. However, a few researchers still doubt HIV is the agent of AIDS. One of their arguments is that Kaposi's sarcoma has occurred, though rarely, in young gay men with no sign of immunodeficiency. As noted in Chapter 4, recent evidence indicates that a newly discovered virus, sexually transmissible but unrelated to HIV, may be involved in KS. And while KS can occur without HIV, it clearly runs a much more aggressive course in HIV-positive people.

Based on the linear progression of AIDS development, we can now extrapolate that about 95 percent of homosexual men infected with HIV-1 will eventually develop AIDS. Their symptom-free period will vary according to a bell-shaped curve (Figure 1.1). Very few individuals will develop AIDS in the first year after infection or in the "last" year, projected to be fifteen to twenty years after infection. Most people will progress to AIDS after an average asymptomatic period of about ten years.

The data suggest that our two nonprogressors remain well not because of virus variation but because of host variation. In other words, these men did not get an unusually weak virus but are, for some reason, unusually well defended hosts. All of us are genetically programmed to offer a more or less effective immune response to HIV and other invaders. The response to any invader involves many factors, all of which can vary. With HIV, an important variation is seen in the cells that carry the CD4 molecule. From person to person, these cells are more or less hospitable to HIV access, entry, and multiplication. Our two AIDS-free subjects have maintained extremely low levels of circulating virus since their initial infection. In contrast, subjects who have developed AIDS quickly have had extremely high levels during the entire period. Naturally, we are looking hard for the precise factor that seems to protect the nonprogressors.

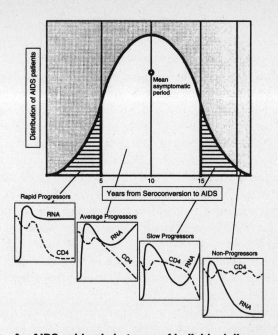

Figure 1.1 **An AIDS epidemic in terms of individual disease and virus level.** *Once HIV-1 invades a given population, the first few AIDS cases appear in six to twelve months. They represent rapid progressors, about 5 percent of the infected population, who suffer immunodeficiency almost from the moment of infection. After seroconversion, they suffer large and incessant amounts of virus, detected as circulating HIV RNA. As shown far left, the RNA drops from its peak, resulting in brief recovery of CD4+ cells, then persists at a high level while CD4+ cells plummet. However, most individuals are average progressors, remaining healthy for five to fifteen years as their body effectively fights the virus. The initially high RNA drops farther and for a longer time than in the first group, and CD4+ cells fall more gradually. These people become ill only when the virus finally breaks through and rises again. About 5 to 10 percent of infected individuals are slow progressors who stay healthy longer than 15 years. The RNA drops significantly as CD4+ cells resist decline. Only when the virus changes to become more aggressive can it rise and cause disease. Marked by clumped cells, this change can occur in all groups but is notably late in this group. In the end, less than 1 percent of infected people are nonprogressors. They remain well so long that their HIV risk is finally overtaken by their risk of cancer or heart disease. As shown far right, the RNA drops steeply and never recovers, while CD4+ cells stay high. Nonprogression may be linked to a crippled HIV, unusually resistant CD4+ cells, excellent HIV-1 immunity, or some combination of these factors. (Hogervorst et al. 1995; Jurriaans et al. 1994.)*

More clues to virus and host variation can be found by comparing HIV and AIDS in the three major risk groups: homosexual men, IV drug users, and hemophiliacs. All three groups are susceptible to HIV-1, but they differ in their AIDS frequency rates and their length of symptom-free periods. AIDS occurs at a somewhat higher rate among gay men than among IV drug users and hemophiliacs, even though the sexual transmission of HIV is far less efficient than its transmission by injection.

For IV drug users and hemophiliacs, certain host factors are known to lower AIDS frequency and lengthen the symptom-free period. All other things being equal, the younger a hemophiliac, the better his defense against AIDS. As for drug users, the frequent sharing of syringes means frequent exposure to HIV. However, once infected, they derive a small benefit from this dangerous practice. The constant injection of foreign blood seems to dull or confuse the immune response, leading to cell *anergy* (the opposite of *energy*), which slightly curbs reproduction of the CD4+ cells. This, in turn, slightly curbs multiplication of HIV, since the virus depends on host reproductive mechanisms.

Much evidence indicates that host factors, more than virus factors, are responsible when HIV is thwarted; conversely, host factors are less responsible when the virus thrives. All HIVs seem to be viable and virulent, and some have found ways to increase their damage. For example, some HIV-1 strains seem able to change their envelope to facilitate entry into CD4+ cells. They can also mutate the genes that regulate their multiplication, to step up the rate. So HIV needs no help from a weak defense, but apparently it can be slowed by a strong defense. One may say that increases in the rate of disease progression are more virus-dependent, while decreases are more host-dependent.

If all known HIV types have gained the virulence to cause AIDS and death, is this virulence now increasing or decreasing? Does the HIV of the Western epidemic cause AIDS faster now than in the early 1980s? Preliminary evidence is discouraging at first glance. A collaborative study of homosexual groups in San Francisco, New York, and Amsterdam showed that men infected during the first five years of the epidemic remained healthy longer than those infected during the second five years. This suggests that HIV virulence had increased in these gay communities.

The good news is that virulence seems to have dropped slightly since then (Figure 1.2). Of course, even the fastest acting AIDS usually takes four to six years to develop, so most Amsterdam men in our first five-year group were infected soon after HIV entered the community in 1980. The

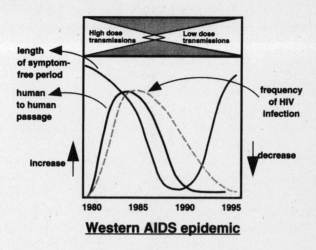

Western AIDS epidemic

Figure 1.2 **The link between rapidity of spread and HIV incidence and virulence.** *Early in the Western AIDS epidemic, the Amsterdam gay community saw frequent HIV transmission events (unprotected anogenital sex) and rapid human-to-human passage linked to a marked increase in newly infected people. HIV virulence also increased because the transmissions occurred when donors had high virus loads, so recipients received large populations. The dominant strains decreased the length of the average symptom-free period and hastened disease. A turning point was reached when a safe sex campaign reduced the number of sex partners and high-risk acts. After 1985, slower passage of HIV resulted in fewer new infections and declining virulence. Aggressive viruses ceased to dominate as they died with rapid progressors. These factors lengthened the average symptom-free period and produced a somewhat less aggressive epidemic with a higher proportion of slow or nonprogressor viruses.* (Keet et al. in press; Veugelers et al. 1994.)

second five-year group was infected in the mideighties, at the peak of sexual activity and HIV infection among Amsterdam homosexuals. Since that high point of 1984–1985, when HIV incidence (i.e., new infections) was 8 percent, the incidence among these men has steadily declined. It had dropped below 1 percent in 1993. Over this same period, HIV circulation has decreased along with high-risk sex. Because of educational programs and other factors, many gay men in Amsterdam have reduced the number of their sex partners and their episodes of unprotected anogenital contact.

Both types of reduction lower the risk, but particularly the latter. Whether sex is homosexual or heterosexual, the probability of acquiring HIV-1 is related less to promiscuity than to the type of contact and the sex of the partner. Especially among men who have sex with men, the number of partners is far less important than the kind of sex they practice.

The most dangerous sex is anogenital: anal penetration by the penis. The more often an uninfected man is anally penetrated by a man infected with HIV-1, the greater his chance of acquiring HIV and AIDS, whether his partners are few or many. Limited studies of heterosexual couples in Africa suggest a parallel, at least with regard to some HIV-1 strains. That is, the more frequently an uninfected woman is anally penetrated by a seropositive man, the greater her risk, whether the situation is monogamous or polygamous.

The safest sex is that between two women, even if they engage in anal stimulation. In fact, two women engaged in such contact (i.e., nonpenile but involving some kind of penetration) are at less risk than two men engaged in the same type of contact, possibly because force is less often a factor. The more forceful the anal penetration, the more likely it is to cause lesions, which invite infection.

We are very encouraged to see that safer sex may have reduced not only new HIV infections but HIV virulence in Amsterdam. Preliminary data from our Amsterdam cohort studies show that men newly infected when circulation had dropped (from 1989 to 1993) are progressing more slowly to AIDS than men infected when HIV circulation was highest (from 1984 to 1988).

Much evidence suggests that HIV virulence, or damage, is directly related to its rate of circulation. This is because the virus load needed for efficient HIV transmission depends on virus reproduction within host cells that are crucial to host well-being. As already noted, the faster and more often HIV changes hosts, the more deadly it becomes. Our own studies have shown that the virus is more aggressive in times of rapid spread and less aggressive when spread is relatively slow. Spread depends on two factors: the opportunity to transmit HIV and the infectivity of the virus. Opportunity depends on the frequency of the transmission event, whether it is unprotected sex, blood transfusion, or IV drug use. Infectivity depends on the level or amount of virus in the transmitting fluid as well as the susceptibility of the host cells to that particular virus.

Looking at sexual transmission (by far the most common of the three routes), we have seen that virtually all newly infected individuals have high virus loads during the first few months (Figure 1.1). As measured by the HIV RNA in their blood, they have about equal amounts of circulating virions, making them equally HIV-infectious. But soon a distinction develops between progressors and nonprogressors (i.e., those rapidly progressing to AIDS and those progressing slowly or not at all). The progressors are highly infectious due to persistent high virus loads in all their body fluids. They transmit a highly aggressive virus that reproduces fast and sustains high levels in its next host. However, progressors are highly infectious for a relatively short time due to rapid disease progression. As their CD4+ cells fall, their sexual activity tends to decline because they feel increasingly ill and develop unattractive symptoms: the dark red Kaposi lesions, the continual cough of *P. carinii* pneumonia, or devastating diarrhea.

In contrast, the nonprogressors are less infectious for a relatively long time because the virus load declines in their fluids. As their immune systems keep AIDS at bay, they feel healthy enough to continue sexual activity, but they transmit a weaker virus. It reproduces relatively slowly and cannot sustain high levels in the next host. Of course, as the epidemic continues, the progressors with their aggressive HIV contribute less and less to the viral mix. They drop out of sexual activity and ultimately die. Therefore, we see that a new AIDS epidemic is dominated by the more infectious virus of progressors, but a late-stage epidemic is dominated by the weaker virus of nonprogressors.

At times of high spread, the stronger virus shrinks the average symptom-free period because it needs less time to break down the immune system. At times of low spread, the weaker virus leads to a longer average symptom-free period. We have compelling evidence that breakdown occurs faster when HIV is acquired (by any route) from an AIDS patient whose symptom-free period was relatively short.

These observations are based on various studies but particularly on our own work in Amsterdam. This has involved a highly active subgroup of relatively young gay men whose sexual habits—and the spread of HIV in their community—have changed rapidly over a short period. Although many gay men have stable long-term relationships, this highly active subgroup combines youthful potency with militant expression of emancipated homosexuality. Their motivation is understandable, but their frequent and anonymous sexual contacts (sometimes several in a day, or several hundred in a year) have given the Western HIV a golden opportunity. At times of high spread, the virus may be introduced by one man to another who, the same day or soon after, conveys it to a third man, and so on. In New York, one man was simultaneously infected with two HIV strains by two different partners within just a few days.

Such promiscuity, practiced routinely throughout a good-sized community, may be unprecedented in history. It may be approximated by heterosexual men who continually visit many different prostitutes, but such men are rare, as far as we can tell. For one thing, prostitutes cost money. In contrast, gay encounters in bathrooms and bathhouses are largely free of charge. It is a tragic accident that HIV-1 was introduced to a population where such activity—so perfectly suited to its passage!—had become the hallmark of liberation. This first HIV epidemic got off to a very good start.

Fortunately, as shown in Amsterdam, preventive measures can reduce HIV infections and actually reverse the spiral of aggressive infection. Fewer people get HIV and AIDS. They stay healthier longer because the virus is weaker and gives them a longer symptom-free period.

However, HIV remains. Now that it has found us, we are locked in a dynamic relationship with this virus. We have seen the benefits of lower HIV circulation, but to sustain those benefits a population such as the Amsterdam gay community must keep the dangers in mind. Members of such a community need to know that they can take control and reduce the threat. Then, having done so, they must remain on guard. If they feel more healthy, see less illness and death, forget the risk, and return to risky behavior, they will quickly revive the threat. To keep HIV in check, everyone who is sexually active—gay or straight—must avoid the high-risk behavior that gives HIV the advantage.

If the virulence of HIV fluctuates with its level of circulation, what does this mean for the worldwide future of AIDS? An infection, harmful or not, can pass through three stages: sporadic, epidemic, and endemic. A sporadic infection makes a scattered appearance and may disappear without ever becoming widespread—or it may progress to the second or third stage. The words *epidemic* and *endemic*, like *democracy*, are based on Greek *demos*, "people" or "region." The prefix *epi-* means "over, on top of," so an *epidemic* spreads over an area. The prefix *en-* means "inside of," so *endemic* implies deep roots. An epidemic infection may eventually disappear—but it may progress and become endemic, like cholera in India. Once endemic, it is part of the landscape and is very hard to eradicate although disease, if any, may actually be milder than when the infection was sporadic or epidemic. (While *epidemic, endemic,* and *population* began as human terms, this book will follow general usage and apply them also to nonhumans, avoiding such animal-specific terms as *epizootic* and *enzootic.*)

In North America and Europe, AIDS is epidemic but seems to be holding, and HIV-1 incidence has dropped (Figure 1.3). In South America and Asia, the disease is fast reaching epidemic proportions. It could easily become endemic because of factors such as poor education, communication, and medical care, which have already made it near endemic in much of Africa. HIV incidence is rising in South America, Asia, and Africa. Several HIV types and subtypes are involved, but if the whole HIV family thrives on circulation, we must expect increasing virulence everywhere, especially in relatively deprived areas.

Since the HIV-1 subtype circulating in North America and Europe is already quite deadly (killing more than 90 percent of its victims within fifteen years), one might ask how it—or other HIVs—could become even more deadly. Evidence suggests that it could kill faster. It could shorten the symptom-free period that follows the initial acute infection. If so, instead of developing AIDS over several years, people might develop the disease in a matter of months. We would then see many millions more cases of AIDS than are projected on the basis of today's average disease-free period.

At this time a very small fraction of infected individuals develop AIDS less than one year after infection. But this could change, as shown by studies of monkeys. Many African monkeys carry a virus closely related to HIV. By analogy, it is called *simian immunodeficiency virus* (SIV), though it does absolutely no harm to its African monkey hosts. However, it harms Asian monkeys. This was discovered when African and Asian monkeys, imported to the United States for laboratory use, were housed together. Suddenly the Asian monkeys contracted a fatal AIDS-like disease. Researchers later found that certain SIV strains could kill Asian monkeys in as little as several weeks or months. These lethal strains had been developed in the laboratory by rapid passaging through many monkeys: SIV-infected blood from one monkey was injected into another, whose infected blood was injected into another, and so on.

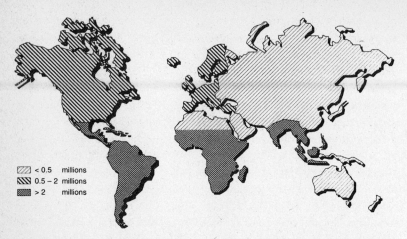

Figure 1.3   Worldwide distribution of 18.5 million adult HIV-1 infections, 1980 to 1995. *HIV-1 infection is still rising in Africa, Asia, and South America. It is somewhat declining in the United States and Europe while shifting from gay communities via IV drug users to the inner-city poor. In Europe this shift is strongest in countries of Eastern Europe. Wherever the epidemic started, it now plagues the most deprived areas of the world.*

Could this kind of virulence develop among humans? Outside Europe and North America, AIDS spreads mainly by heterosexual relations, perinatal infection, and contaminated blood and hospital supplies. Control strategies must aim to safeguard the blood supplies and hospital equipment. But if HIV thrives on rapidity of consecutive transmission, these strategies will not be enough. Somehow people in Africa, Asia, and South America must be educated to lower their number of sexual partners and, even more important, their high-risk sex acts. Gay men in Amsterdam and other areas have shown this can be done. Other strategies will be described later in this book.

Even in North America and Europe, where HIV incidence is dropping, we cannot rest easy. The decreased incidence may lead to decreased virulence and even to a weakened or attenuated virus. But virulence could just as well be boosted by ominous changes in the Western epidemic. At first HIV-1 was spread mainly by homosexual relations, then by needle sharing among drug users. Now it is infecting more women and children, most of whom have no direct connection with drugs or homosexuals. HIV infection is seen mainly among the poor and homeless in big cities like New York, but it could easily become a more general threat. The Western epidemic, like those elsewhere, could gain momentum by spreading heterosexually as well as homosexually.

Ultimately HIV is a threat to us all, everywhere in the world. We can all agree that something must be done, but how do we disarm this virus that disarms us so well? How can we render it less aggressive, even harmless?

Nature and science will ultimately show us the way, but two promising avenues have so far been disappointing. The first involves searching the HIV family for types that are relatively harmless, either because of inherently low infectivity or loss of infectivity (attenuation). Such relatively weak viruses could give insight into more harmful types. They might even protect us against them, as cowpox was used by Jenner to protect against smallpox.

At this point, we have discovered and studied two possibilities that will later be discussed in depth. The first is HIV type 2 (HIV-2), which emerged in the West African interior. This virus causes AIDS, but very slowly and with lower frequency than HIV-1. HIV-2 is mainly confined to West Africa, where HIV-1 subtypes are appearing with increasing frequency. More time and study are needed to tell how well HIV-2 infection protects people against HIV-1. Although most West African AIDS victims harbor only one of the two viruses, a rare few harbor both. This could mean HIV-2 offers incomplete or temporary protection. However, with a double infection we cannot yet tell whether the two viruses entered simultaneously or, if sequentially, which came first. We can still hope that HIV-2 has some protective potential, and new data point tentatively in that direction.

Meanwhile, HIV-1 is overtaking the slower HIV-2 in West Africa, but HIV-2 is not likely to disappear. It has a proven monkey reservoir or home base: the sooty mangabey. This monkey comfortably hosts an SIV that becomes HIV-2 when transmitted to the human body. Such transmission has been documented on several occasions. It may even occur quite frequently, as when monkeys bite—or are eaten by—humans.

The other new type to be studied is HIV type 0 (HIV-0). It was discovered in 1990 by Belgian researchers Guido van der Groen and Peter Piot, who initially thought they had found HIV-3. Their virus seemed unrelated to HIV-2, which was discovered in 1985 by François Clavel, Luc Montagnier, and colleagues. It also seemed unrelated to HIV-1 but is now considered a distantly related HIV-1 subgroup. Some have called it "O" for "outgroup," but "zero" is now preferred. Originally found only in Cameroon and Gabon, HIV-0 was isolated from several AIDS patients by different researchers, leaving no doubt that it can cause the disease in humans. Its virulence is unknown, but its spread is extremely limited. The virus has just recently been seen in Europe, mainly France, in a handful of immigrants from Cameroon and Gabon. In Africa, it is only rarely seen outside its accustomed area. Even there, HIV-0 occurs in much less than 10 percent of AIDS victims. The rest are infected with the more common HIV-1 subtypes.

As with HIV-2, the closest relative to HIV-0 is not another human AIDS virus but a monkey virus. Found in chimpanzees, it is called *chimpanzee immunodeficiency virus* (CIV) or, more often, SIV cpz. Like other SIVs, it does not harm its natural host. Very few chimpanzees in the wild seem to harbor this virus, but its transmission to a human has occurred at least once, and maybe more.

While HIV-2 and HIV-0 have great research value, they are not too promising as barriers against HIV-1. Though they spread and act slowly, they still cause AIDS. As long as an HIV type destroys our defense system, it is a deadly virus sooner or later. We want one that will protect us while causing little or no immunodisturbance—but perhaps no in-between exists for HIV. This virus may have evolved so that its multiplication in humans always decimates the immune cells to a fatal degree. In fact, one might question whether HIV-0 and HIV-2 are that different from HIV-1. Perhaps they are only in different equilibrium with their host populations, most likely because of host factors such as sexual partner rates.

Our second avenue is to find a virus outside the HIV family: something similar but harmless to its natural host. We have already found CIV, other SIVs, and even analogs beyond the primate family. As discussed in later chapters, these viruses offer tantalizing clues to the HIV family. But so far, none offers us protection from HIV. Although closely related to the killer, these viruses are remarkable in that they never cause the slightest harm to their natural hosts. SIVs can even move among various types of African monkeys without harm. In fact, they seem to inhabit a different virus world than our HIV. Without knowing the terrible AIDS story, we would never believe that these innocent monkey viruses could kill. Yet they kill humans, and some of them kill Asian monkeys.

What makes these simian viruses perfectly harmless to some primates and deadly to others? How can they be so well adapted to multiply in human immune cells? Since we find no harmless HIVs, it appears that SIV just naturally develops into an AIDS-causing pathogen after roaming from human to human for a number of viral generations.

2

The Rise of the Western AIDS Epidemic

When AIDS emerged as an epidemic in the early 1980s, researchers scrambled to identify the virus and develop tests to diagnose infection and monitor world blood supplies. They also scrambled to trace the disease to its probable source by combing earlier medical literature and investigating old cases. Some brilliant work was done, but mistakes were made because of pressure, new techniques, and some prejudices. A crucial error in identification would go undiscovered for years, causing confusion and hampering progress.

The story of this error begins at the Institut Pasteur, where Françoise Barré-Sinoussi, Jean-Claude Chermann, and Luc Montagnier found the first AIDS virus. Its activity was detected in the lymph node of a young gay man who was given the code name "Bru." He was infected but had not yet developed AIDS, a point that turned out to be very important.

The Pasteur group ran into trouble when it tried to grow and isolate the virus. Some organisms grow like weeds, but others must be coaxed like orchids. The process can be especially tricky with a little-known organism, but a standard procedure is followed. On nutrient medium, a bit of fluid or tissue thought to contain the organism is grown, or cultured, with live cells that are uninfected but infectable. Various media are used to encourage various types of organisms. The live cells are commonly human or animal skin cells, but in the case of HIV they are CD4+ white blood cells. Most cultivation is *in vitro,* "in glass" (e.g., a flask or petri dish) but can also be *in vivo,* "in a living system" (e.g., a laboratory animal). With proper temperature and other conditions, the desired organism multiplies and, in this case, infects the live cells. The organism can then be seen and studied. Ideally, it can also be isolated, or recovered, from the culture by means of various filtration and purification techniques.

The Bru lymph node was first cultured in early January 1983 and, on January 15, it shed an enzyme absolutely unique to the lentivirus group (from Latin *lentus,* "slow"). Now called HIV-1 Bru, the virus was initially called JBB/LAV: Bru's initials plus an acronym for lymphadenovirus, or lymph node virus. The Bru virus grew slowly and with difficulty, but its identity and activity were reported in the May 20, 1983, issue of *Science.*

The Pasteur group was widely acclaimed but very worried. In the world of virology, finding a new virus is not enough: you must propagate and isolate the organism for analysis by other virologists. The French had not yet isolated their new lentivirus and, since it proved hard to grow, they feared they might lose it. On June 26 they started a second Bru culture (JBB2/LAV). In July, Montagnier sent a sample of this second culture to Bob Gallo of the US National Cancer Institute (NCI) in Bethesda, Maryland. That same month, Chermann sent DNA from the virus to Beatrice Hahn and Flossie Wong-Staal, then working with Gallo. The virus did not thrive in Gallo's laboratory, and the DNA was never analyzed.

However, the French had found a similar virus in a man who already had AIDS. On June 9 Barré-Sinoussi began to culture this second virus, code-named "Lai." It grew much faster than Bru and also grew on permanent cell lines—cells made immortal by various techniques—whereas the Bru virus grew only on primary cells. Everybody was delighted because virologists have a prejudice for fast-growing viruses and for viruses that grow on cell lines. Viruses that grow on primary cells are much less convenient for two reasons. First, primary cells come from living donors, who must provide them every few days. Second, primary cells produce virus only temporarily because they quickly die, especially after infection with HIV.

Virologists also like viruses grown on cell lines because they produce continuously and can therefore be studied better. In fact, many organisms thrive on cell lines that would never grow on the corresponding primary cells in vitro or in vivo. For example, a feline virus might infect a human cell line but never actually infect a person in the real world. Naturally, the virologists working with HIV especially wanted good production because of the need for HIV antibody tests to diagnose infected individuals and monitor blood supplies.

On July 20 Barré-Sinoussi prepared to culture both Bru and Lai again. For only the first or second time, she would use new cocultivation techniques developed in late June or early July. Designed to maintain a cell-killing virus, this protocol involved addition of growth factors and fresh activated lymphocytes at the beginning of the culture and throughout the process. So Barré-Sinoussi collected fresh CD4+ cells and divided them between two flasks. Then she added a Bru sample to one flask and a Lai sample to the other. As before, Lai grew in five days, but, surprisingly, Bru grew in nine days instead of the twelve days it had previously required. Not only that, but this Bru was found later to grow in cell lines.

Unfortunately, it was also found—much later—that the Lai culture had somehow contaminated the Bru culture. The Bru strain of virus grew well because it was being overtaken by the more active Lai strain. Labeled JBB2'/LAV, the mixed culture was sent for analysis to Gallo in September 1983 and to Robin Weiss, in London, in February 1984. Nobody knew it was actually Bru/Lai bearing the pseudonym of Bru. The original Bru virus that remained at Pasteur was forgotten in a lab freezer until controversy arose, eight years later, as to who had isolated the very first HIV strain. Until then, the Bru virus, which everybody thought they were using for research and development of HIV tests, was never used by anybody for any purpose.

This case of mistaken identity, beginning with contamination of Bru, may seem impossible to people who imagine that all researchers are highly organized people who work in spotless laboratories. In reality, researchers range between this orderly stereotype and that of the "mad scientist." Like other work, science is often disorderly, especially at times of crisis. At the most serene times, people put many little samples in many big lab freezers, and things can get lost. When a sample is cultured, it can easily be contaminated in many ways: by another organism under study (as in this case), by an organism in the air, or by skin cells sloughed by a researcher. Contamination is a constant and growing factor in laboratory work, especially when the work involves new materials or protocols. Increasingly fine detection techniques reveal contamination or "background noise" that nobody could detect only a few years ago. Formerly invisible viruses can now be readily seen in a culture, and mistakenly diagnosed as a new organism. The best scientists are very careful, but they know that awareness of contamination—its ubiquity and inevitability—is even more important than being careful.

The switch of two strains of the same virus subtype might make little difference in some cases. However, the exchange of Lai for Bru was a virological horror story. The real Bru was a much better prototype of the HIV causing the Western epidemic than was the Lai virus masquerading as Bru. Today we know that virus from seropositive but still healthy individuals (like the man who gave us Bru) tends to grow *only* on primary cells, not on permanent cell lines. In about 50 percent of HIV-infected individuals, a change occurs that can easily be seen in the laboratory. As much as one or two years before AIDS develops, the virus suddenly grows very rapidly and makes blood cells clump to form giant syncytial cells. (Greek *syn,* "with" plus *cyte,* "cell," describes the conglomeration.) The virus is then much more transmissible to permanent cell lines. However, many scientists believe the virus at that stage is much *less* transmissible among actual human beings, if only because health and sexual activity begin to decline. The virus has less chance for transmission and, if transmitted, appears more likely to be defeated by the immune defense of its new host.

So a virus at the Lai stage rarely circulates and is less infectious than a virus like Bru. Virologists who were studying Lai (misnamed Bru), thriving on permanent cell lines, would have learned far more about HIV-1 and AIDS from the real Bru, despite its culture difficulties. They were like the man in the joke, looking for his keys under a streetlight: he hadn't lost them there, but the light was good.

The fact that the HIV strains conveniently growing on cell lines had little to do with the spread of the HIV epidemic did not dawn on anyone for quite a long time. After three years, Brigitta Åsjö and Eva-Maria Fenyö of the Karolinska Institute in Sweden discovered the important biological distinction between slow/low HIV and rapid/high HIV. The slow HIV is found in 95 percent of people newly infected with the virus. The fast HIV is found in only 5 percent of people newly infected but in about 50 percent of those who have progressed to AIDS. The slow/low and rapid/high designations describe HIV strains according to their speed and level of growth in culture. Unfortunately, the Åsjö-Fenyö discovery was not generally known or used to unmask Lai as an imposter.

So for several years we learned more than we needed to know about one virus (Lai) and nothing at all about the virus we really cared about (Bru).

The virologists' preference for strains grown on cell lines caused confusion and would lead to controversy between Gallo and Montagnier.

We must now backtrack to late 1983 and early 1984, when the mixed Bru-Lai samples (mislabled JBB2'/LAV) were sent to Gallo in the United States and Weiss in England. Both groups had heard that Bru was hard to grow on cell lines. However, they attempted this feat, and, of course, they succeeded. What they never guessed was that, by doing this, they both—simultaneously—completed the switch from Bru to Lai. In their laboratories, Lai quickly overgrew and obliterated Bru, and the researchers began to propagate and study the wrong strain.

At this time the Gallo group was growing other viruses, seeking to identify the first truly US strain of HIV. This would cause problems, especially since the researchers proceeded in a strange way. On November 15, 1983, Mika Popovic pooled the cultures of various HIVs of US origin. Then on January 2, 1984, he added cultures from seven more US individuals, all from groups at high risk for AIDS. Meanwhile, he was doing work on the French virus. In February, by some miracle, he isolated Lai virus from the pooled US samples! Of course, the French culture had contaminated the US samples, but Popovic mistook Lai for a new strain. He inoculated it onto the permanent human T-cell line H9 (Hut 78) and began producing HIV-1 Lai, which he named HIV-1 IIIB.

As late as 1994, Luc Montagnier and anybody who received his virus samples was working not with HIV-1 Bru but with HIV-1 Lai without knowing it. Similarly, Bob Gallo and anybody who used his virus samples was working not with HIV-1 IIIB but, again, with HIV-1 Lai.

The final irony is that, not only was HIV-1 Lai going under two pseudonyms, but it never actually infected the man for whom it was named. The virus that everyone was using had undergone genetic mutations and was no longer the strain isolated at Pasteur. It had become an unusual strain that has never infected anyone by the normal routes of HIV transmission. Except for three workers infected in the laboratory, it has infected only lab cultures. Yet this odd strain was long used to generate HIV antibodies for tests to diagnose newly infected people and monitor our blood supplies. These tests were extremely useful but were probably less sensitive than optimum.

Both Montagnier and Gallo were responsible for contaminations. However, the French had the good luck to contaminate their cultures with their own virus, while the Americans had the bad luck to contaminate their cultures with someone else's virus. Apparently, the US strains pooled by

Popovic all had slow growth characteristics. They could not be adapted to cell lines, which allowed Lai to stand out. But in late 1983 the Gallo group succeeded in growing a Haitian isolate, HIV-1 RF, on a permanent cell line. In 1984, the group repeated this coup with HIV-1 MN, an isolate from a child infected in Newark, New Jersey. Then Jay Levy of the University of California, San Francisco, isolated several US strains of HIV-1 from homosexual men living in the San Francisco area.

Gallo's HIV-1 MN strain from Newark would become very important. It was found among samples drawn from several children born to mothers with AIDS or at risk for AIDS. MN was born October 1980 to an IV drug–using mother. (His initials were changed to protect his identity.) When about one year old, the boy started to bleed internally due to the shortage of platelets that often accompanies HIV infection. The shortage is caused mainly by destruction of platelets in the spleen so, according to common procedure, the boy's spleen was removed. This was done in 1984, when MN had yet to show any immunological abnormalities or signs of AIDS. His spleen tissue was sent to Gallo's laboratory, and a virus was recovered from the cultured cells. Surprisingly, it was found to grow readily on cell lines and, unlike Lai, to resemble closely the average HIV strain circulating among infected gay men and IV drug users in Europe and the United States. So the virological horror story had at least one happy ending.

To review, see Figure 2.1. Montagnier found a virus (JBB/LAV, later HIV-1 Bru) that was very representative of viruses causing the AIDS epidemic in the United States and Europe. Then he lost it. He unwittingly replaced it with a second virus, HIV-1 Lai. Neither Gallo nor Weiss discovered the switch but instead got Montagnier's second virus to grow in cell lines. Years later, Gallo was accused of stealing Montagnier's first virus (Bru) and claiming credit for its discovery. But to everyone's chagrin, including his own, Gallo himself found that HIV-1 IIIB was actually Lai and bore no resemblance to the original Bru strain. (Remember, he had received the original Bru in July 1983 but could not grow it. He had received more Bru in September, but it was contaminated and ultimately overtaken by Lai.) It was Lai that Popovic succeeded in growing on permanent cell lines. It was Lai that contaminated the pooled culture from which Popovic hoped to recover the first specifically US HIV-1 strain. It was Lai that went to several pharmaceutical companies for production of HIV antibody tests. Then, in 1984, Gallo's laboratory isolated HIV-1 MN.

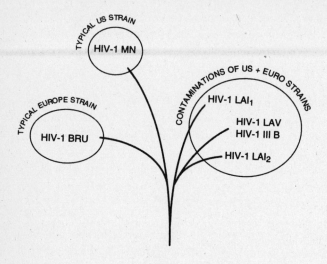

Figure 2.1 Family tree of first US and European HIV-1 isolates. *HIV-1 Bru was the first strain to be isolated. Recovered by the team at the Institut Pasteur, it can be considered the prototype European HIV-1. Its US counterpart, HIV-1 MN, was isolated in Bethesda, Maryland, by the team of the National Cancer Institute. HIV-1 Lai, HIV-IIIB, and LAV are all descendants of a French strain that contaminated cultures on both sides of the Atlantic.* (Lukashov and Goudsmit 1995.)

But which of the two isolates, the French HIV-1 Lai or the American HIV-1 MN, was the most typical of the virus population ravaging the Western world? The definitive answer came between 1987 and 1990, when serological and molecular methods were developed to detect the "signature" of virus strains. As will be detailed in Chapter 3, a feature of the virus envelope is clearly distinctive for most strains. By comparing this feature among many strains, we found that those closely related to HIV-1 MN constituted more than 95 percent of the viruses recovered from HIV-infected people in the United States and Europe, whether they were merely seropositive or had actually developed AIDS. Lai was not found in a single person.

In the end, Montagnier and Gallo each won "first prize." The French isolated the first AIDS virus ever (HIV-1 Lai), and the Americans isolated the first virus that was truly representative of the Western AIDS epidemic (HIV-1 MN). The original Bru was even more representative, due to its slow-growing properties, but nobody—not even Montagnier—realized this virus existed until years later.

Where Was HIV before 1980?

While Montagnier and Gallo were making their landmark discoveries, other researchers were tracing the history of HIV and AIDS with surprising results. Their main question was, Where was HIV-1 before it emerged among gay men in the early 1980s? Before it launched this epidemic, the virus must have caused sporadic cases that went unnoticed because they were rare or seldom lethal, or both. Were these cases sufficiently puzzling that physicians had reported them in various journals? Could we pick up a trail of such reports and follow it, case by case, to discover when and where HIV was first introduced? Since 1980, researchers have been looking for these signposts. The older literature is well indexed (if not computerized), but one cannot look up AIDS, HIV, or even immunodeficiency. One must look for cases of *P. carinii* pneumonia (PCP) and other odd infections. The search is slow and probably incomplete, but an intriguing picture can now be pieced together.

Most people assume that the AIDS epidemic originated in large US cities with extensive homosexual populations, like New York and San Francisco, and then moved to European cities like Amsterdam and Copenhagen by way of American homosexuals or by European homosexuals infected in America. However, it now looks as if the first AIDS victims were Europeans who had never been to America or encountered American homosexuals. The most compelling cases involve two sailors, one from Norway and one from England.

The Norwegian sailor had traveled extensively not only in Europe but in Africa, where he could have met HIV. He was infected sometime before 1966, when he was seen with persistent enlargement of the lymph nodes. In 1971 a sample was taken that much later, using Lai reagents in the mid-1980s, showed he was seropositive for HIV. This sample and many others pivotal to the AIDS story had luckily been frozen. Using technologies available since World War II, many scientists routinely preserve intriguing sera (in a lab freezer) or cells (in liquid nitrogen) for future reference and study.

The Norwegian sailor died in April 1976 from pneumonia, dementia, and other severe neurological abnormalities. He had infected his wife, who died eight months after her husband with similar signs and symptoms. A child born to the couple in 1967 developed generalized candida infection at age two and died in January 1976 of a generalized chicken pox infection. (An infection is generalized when it is not localized to one particular organ or system.) As with the sailor, retrospective serological testing in the mid-1980s showed both mother and child to be HIV-positive. Most likely the child was infected perinatally by the mother.

This sad family history suggests the sailor was infected before 1966 and infected his wife before 1967. If so, HIV was present in Europe by the mid-1960s, if only in this one family. The virus had become strong enough to cause AIDS and was transmissible sexually and perinatally. Recently retrospective serological and molecular evidence suggested that HIV-0 infected the Norwegian sailor and his family.

The second sailor is even more mysterious. When he died in 1959, in Manchester, England, a local pathologist performed an autopsy. He found *P. carinii* and cytomegalovirus in the sailor's lungs, and herpesvirus in and around his anus (Williams, 1960). Years later, after AIDS had been recognized, this same pathologist claimed that his patient—now known as the Manchester sailor—was the first reported case. Studies of frozen tissues from the sailor, preserved by the pathologist, were conducted by virologists in the United Kingdom. They reported finding HIV (Corbitt, 1990), but their results could not be replicated in other studies, notably those conducted by the laboratory of David Ho at the Aaron Diamond AIDS Research Center in New York. Using primers able to trace current varieties of HIV, the Ho group showed that the UK studies were most likely contaminated by material from a victim of the current AIDS epidemic. In a letter to *Nature* (April 6, 1995), Ho reported "serious doubts about the authenticity of the 1959 Manchester man as the first documented case of AIDS due to HIV-1 infection." Indeed, Ho's analysis showed that the Manchester man was infected by a strain of virus genetically dissimilar to HIV-1. If the Norway sailor and his family were infected by true HIV in the mid-1960s, then the virus had changed considerably since it had infected the Manchester sailor in the late 1950s. The Norwegian sailor and his family seem to have suffered from AIDS as we know it, whereas the Manchester man had an early or incomplete form of the disease.

This man became seriously ill at age twenty-five in December 1958. He was single, and his sexual orientation is unknown. In 1957, with the Royal Navy, he had sailed to Gibraltar and visited Tangier, in Morocco, which even now has very little HIV or AIDS. That was his only trip beyond the United Kingdom. He rapidly developed shortness of breath, nocturnal sweats, weight loss, fatigue, and fever. Early in 1959, deep and painful ulcerations appeared around his mouth and anus. His physicians also noted "scaly brownish lesions on the skin of his back and shoulders." All these problems worsened despite antibiotic therapy, but hormone treatment temporarily improved his appetite and reduced his fever. In the last month of his life, more infections and ulcers appeared on his fingers, lower lip, and tongue. He died after a progressive illness of less than two years. At death his emaciated body was entirely covered with small skin lesions. At autopsy, cause of death was revealed to be PCP combined with generalized cytomegalovirus (CMV) infection. Like *P. carinii*, CMV is ubiquitous and rarely harmful to humans except when immunodeficiency allows opportunistic infection.

By 1962, thirty-three adult cases of PCP had been reported in the medical literature. In all but one, the disease was fatal. In almost all cases this pneumonia occurred simultaneously with other infections or tumors. The most commonly described infections were generalized CMV, tuberculosis, and cryptococcosis. The tumors were usually leukemias and lymphomas. This picture surely resembles AIDS, but in those days an immunodeficiency could not yet be diagnosed by laboratory means.

Many authors who described these cases in the 1950s and 1960s suspected that some underlying cause made the patients fatally vulnerable to infections that normally are innocent. Scientists of the time thought that such lowered resistance was caused either by prolonged hormone therapies or by underlying malignancy. At the same time, they saw that fatal cases of *P. carinii* infection had occurred without any apparent predisposing condition.

Of the thirty-three cases, twenty-seven (82 percent) were men. About half were in their thirties or forties when they died. All cases seemed sporadic in nature. They were noted mainly in Europe (a few on other continents), but no one suspected that an epidemic was building among young adult males. However, the Norwegian sailor and his family—the only individuals to be confirmed HIV-positive—suggest that HIV was already circulating in the 1960s or even the 1950s. If it killed virtually all of its victims (thirty-two of thirty-three), it had already acquired the ability to cause immunodeficiency with fatal outcome.

If most victims were young single males, this HIV may well have been an early variant of HIV-1 subtype B, the virus that started and still dominates the Western epidemic. HIV-1B is now known to spread through homosexual (i.e., anal) intercourse more easily than any other HIV type or subtype. HIV-1B is particularly adapted to invade a host through cells in the mucous membrane lining of the anus. If it was the main culprit in those thirty-three early cases, it had already evolved this affinity for the anal mucosa.

The evidence seems strong that HIV-1 was among us, waiting only for the opportunity—supplied by the gay emancipation movement of the late 1960s and 1970s—to emerge as the epidemic we know today. The medical literature reveals that, while waiting, it caused small and well-documented epidemics of PCP accompanied by generalized CMV infection in several parts of Europe. As far as we know, the largest epidemic, which struck very young children, emerged just before World War II and lasted about twenty years. It affected only children in their first year of life, only in continental Europe, but thousands of children died.

As shown in Figure 2.2, the first cases were reported in 1939 from the Baltic port city of Danzig, then in Germany (now Gdansk, in Poland). The epidemic then spread to Switzerland in 1941, to Austria in 1942, and to Italy in 1946, primarily to the east and north of the peninsula. By the end of the 1940s, it had reached Finland, Denmark, and Sweden. In Germany itself, the epidemic intensified in the early 1950s. However, although it spread to all corners of the country, it was always most concentrated in the eastern part. Especially in cities like Leipzig, Dresden, and Jena, the fatal cases of PCP reached astonishing numbers. After the 1950s, PCP was increasingly seen in Czechoslovakia and Hungary. In Czechoslovakia alone, five hundred children died of this pneumonia during a five-year period (1951–1956). By the end of the decade, the epidemic had apparently leveled off and, by the early 1960s, it had ceased.

How did this epidemic occur and spread? If its basis was an underlying immunodeficiency caused by an HIV-like virus, why did the parents of affected children show no signs of illness? Why did the young victims suc-

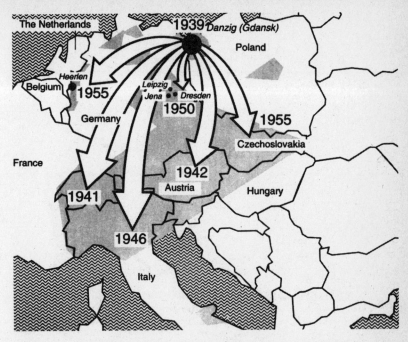

Figure 2.2 **European spread of deadly pneumonia in the 1940s and 1950s**. *This epidemic of pneumocystis pneumonia with CMV infection began with World War II in the Baltic port city of Danzig. It lasted into the 1960s and involved the shaded areas. Adults were affected, but only sporadically. Most infections occurred among newborns of mothers who were uninfected, or at least healthy, suggesting disease transmission by infected fluids or nonsterile needles.* (Koop 1964.)

cumb to acute infection rather than the chronic infection seen today in AIDS patients?

Complete answers are lacking, but partial answers can be found by looking at an isolated and well-described epidemic. It began in 1955 in a single city in the south of the Netherlands: Heerlen in the province of Limburg (Figure 2.3). Except in this one town, PCP occurred only sporadically in the Netherlands both before and after 1955. But in Heerlen, between June 1955 and July 1958, the pneumonia struck eighty-one hospitalized infants, of whom twenty-four died. The whole epidemic was confined to a single unit—the so-called Swedish barrack—of the Kweekschool voor

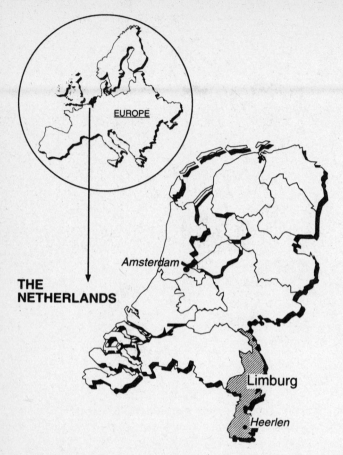

Figure 2.3 **Heerlen, Limburg, the Netherlands**. *Location of PCP and CMV epidemic among newborns 1954–1959.* (Koop 1964.)

Vroedvrouwen, a training hospital for midwives (Figure 2.4a,b,c). After 1948, any newborn born too early or with problems was nursed and treated in the Swedish barrack. Separated from their mothers, such newborns normally stayed in the barrack until they reached a weight of 3,000 grams (about 6 pounds, 10 ounces). The unit accommodated forty to forty-four newborns in seventeen small rooms that had beds for two to four patients.

The population of Limburg was unusual because its coal mines drew miners and their families from beyond the Netherlands, in particular from

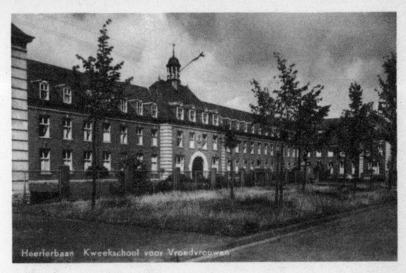

Heerlerbaan Kweekschool voor Vroedvrouwen

Figure 2.4a *The Kweekschool voor Vroedvrouwen, midwife training school, site of the Heerlen epidemic.* (Courtesy of Mrs. E. J. Weyers-Consten)

southeastern and eastern Europe. At the training school for midwives, a high percentage of newborns had been fathered by the foreign miners. Their mothers were often unwed local women, who apparently felt more at ease with the midwives than with medical staff at the local hospital. The PCP epidemic touched only the midwifery school and not the unit for new-borns at nearby St. Joseph's Hospital, even though school and hospital shared the same nurses and pediatricians. Several babies born at the school were transferred to St. Joseph's while very sick with PCP, but they did not start a new chain of infections at the hospital.

Two babies who were born at St. Joseph's died of PCP. They had never been in the barrack but had occupied beds next to transfers from the bar-rack who seemed healthy when they arrived. One of these transfers later developed PCP and died, strengthening the case against the barrack as the origin of infection. A serious search by local general practitioners, hospital physicians, and pathologists found no other local pockets of infection. The epidemic was apparently confined to a single unit in a single hospital in a single Dutch city.

Analysis of all eighty-one PCP cases revealed that the children showed the first signs of disease at minimally about fifty days and maximally one-

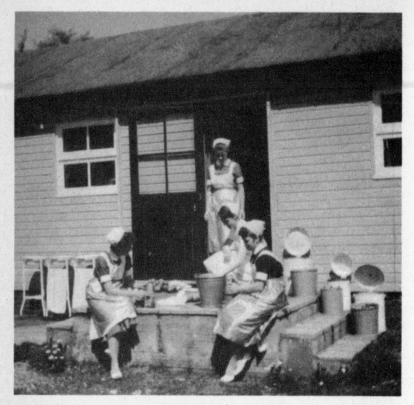

Figure 2.4b   *Nurses with the Swedish barrack in the background.* (Courtesy of Mrs. E. J. Weyers-Consten)

hundred days after birth. The established incubation time for PCP is about one month. Virtually all of us acquire *P. carinii* during our early years, without harm, regardless of our maturity at birth. These facts strongly suggest that in the Limburg epidemic, some cause of diminished immunity was acquired at or soon after birth. This opened the door to *P. carinii* and CMV.

Like *P. carinii*, CMV usually infects us without harm unless it is acquired too early in life. If acquired perinatally, it can cause disease even if immunity is not impaired. When acquired so early, it is usually congenital: it is caught from mothers who carry *P. carinii* and CMV. But normal newborns rarely catch these organisms. Their immune systems protect them until they are old enough to be unharmed by this colonization.

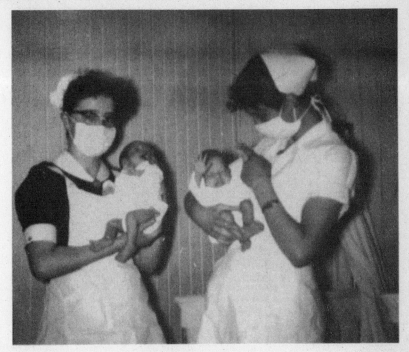

Figure 2.4c   *Nurses with infants.* (Courtesy of Mrs. E. J. Weyers-Consten)

The mothers of newborns in this epidemic showed no manifestations of pneumonia. They did not acquire the cause of immunodeficiency that affected their newborns. The mothers undoubtedly conveyed *P. carinii* and CMV, but what caused immunodeficiency in the newborns? Why did these usually harmless organisms become so deadly? For clues, we must look more closely at the course of the epidemic and its virulence.

First of all, premature birth did not seem to cause the immunodeficiency. During the epidemic, 20 percent of children born prematurely developed PCP, while 15 percent of those born at maturity developed the disease. The five-point difference in percentile cannot be considered meaningful, especially since virtually no cases of PCP were observed in the ward for premature newborns at St. Joseph's Hospital. Besides PCP, the children often had CMV complications. In the laboratory, the most striking observation was a hypergammaglobulinemia. This means an abnormally high level of general antibodies—a sign of chronic infectious disease and a hallmark of AIDS in children (more about pediatric AIDS in a moment).

In 1955, the first year of the epidemic, among 230 admissions to the Swedish barrack there were fourteen cases of PCP and/or CMV: an incidence of 6 percent (Figure 2.5). Of these first fourteen cases, four died: a mortality rate of 29 percent. The following year, 1956, saw only 6 cases of disease among almost as many admissions (229)—a drop to 3 percent—and no fatalities. One would assume that the epidemic was over, but the next two years proved otherwise. In 1957, twenty-eight cases of disease occurred among 194 newborns treated in the barrack, raising the incidence to 14 percent. Simultaneously, the death rate rose to 32 percent of affected infants.

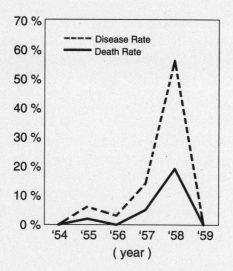

Figure 2.5   **Disease and death rate of newborns at the Swedish barrack, 1954–1959**. *At the height of the epidemic of PCP with CMV infection of the lungs, 56 percent of all infants admitted to the Swedish barrack suffered disease; 19 percent of all admissions died of the disease.* (Koop 1964.)

So the disease had become not only more frequent but more aggressive. In 1958, up to August 1, admissions were only fifty-nine because both parents and doctors began to avoid the deadly barrack. Of these, thirty-three newborns developed disease, a majority of those admitted (56 percent). But while incidence rose, virulence did not change: eleven of the diseased children died, a mortality rate of 33 percent. In April 1958 after three deaths occurred in rapid succession, it was decided to halt new admissions to the barrack. In July 1958 the last newborns left, and immediately thereafter the Swedish barrack was closed forever. No new cases of newborn PCP have occurred in the area since that time.

The highly unusual fatality of the infection strongly points to a preexisting immunodeficiency, that is, a deficiency not caused by premature birth or treatments related to birth. What, then, was special about these children? The only special and consistent factor was their presence in the Swedish barrack. What happened there that did not happen anywhere else?

Injections are said to have been given rarely, but blood transfusions are documented in some children, as well as nikethamide injections to improve breathing, and sometimes antibiotics. Protocols and practice for these treatment interventions must have been largely the same at the midwifery school and St. Joseph's Hospital, since the same staff were involved. But how else can we explain the epidemic except to imagine transmission of immunodeficiency by some contaminated intervention? We have seen this happen more than once in the current AIDS epidemic and in various pediatric epidemics. In the 1980s, small but dramatic epidemics of AIDS occurred among children in several hospitals, orphanages, and childrens' homes of Eastern Europe. They occurred because reusable syringes and needles were not sterilized between injections, and single-use needles and syringes were beyond the budget. In these cases, HIV was spread because the blood of an infected child remained in a syringe that was used to treat an uninfected child.

Another scenario was seen in the Hospital of Leiden University in the Netherlands in 1981. As was customary in those days, premature children receiving intravenous nutrition also received transfusions of plasma. Eleven such children were subsequently found to be infected with HIV, and after ten years of follow-up, eight of them had died. Retrospective analysis revealed that all eleven had received plasma from one individual: a homosexual man who donated blood when he was HIV-positive but had no symptoms.

Either of these two scenarios could have brought HIV to the Limburg newborns. It is difficult to explain why such epidemics occurred in widely separated hospitals of Eastern and Western Europe, with different staff and protocols, but did not occur in St. Joseph's Hospital and the nearby Swedish barrack, with their shared staff and protocols. Still, it is easy to imagine how the virus (if HIV played a role) was carried from Eastern Europe to the Netherlands. Most likely, at least one adult—probably a coal miner from Poland, Czechoslovakia, or Italy—brought the virus to Limburg. This one adult could have died from AIDS with little notice. Like the Norwegian sailor, he could have transmitted the virus to his wife and offspring. His infected wife (or girlfriend) could have given birth in the Swedish barrack to a child who was HIV-positive but seemingly healthy. Unsterilized needles and syringes could have spread the virus from child to child. The less likely scenario, analogous to the Leiden incident, is that a coal miner's HIV-infected blood was used for plasma therapy of newborns. However, no such practice is documented.

The early presence of HIV in Europe seems clear from the sporadic cases of opportunistic infections and tumors (thirty-three documented by 1962), the few cases confirmed HIV-positive (the Norwegian sailor and family), and the epidemics among newborns. These early incarnations of HIV had caused AIDS, but in a strange way. In adults, the 1950s disease looked much like AIDS as we know it today. However, in children the 1950s disease was importantly different from pediatric AIDS as seen since the 1980s. In the earlier time, children sometimes died rapidly after birth—but often they lived and appeared to have *cleared the virus*. Regarding the Limburg cases, we have no reports of recurrence or delayed effect. No children who recovered from early PCP (with or without CMV) died years later of other manifestations of immunodeficiency. No children who escaped PCP, despite barracks exposure, later showed any sign of immunodeficiency.

Therefore, if the agent of those early epidemics was a variant of HIV-1B, one must assume that its biological characteristics have changed in the intervening thirty to forty years. That a virus of the HIV family may once have caused acute and often fatal disease *from which total recovery was possible* is not as unlikely as it sounds. Exactly such a syndrome has been seen in cattle infected with the Jembrana disease virus, which is related to HIV.

Jembrana disease was first noted in cattle on Bali, Indonesia, in 1964. It is an acute and serious disease with a mortality of 15 to 20 percent, much like the disease of the Swedish barrack in Heerlen. Following a short incubation period of five to twelve days, acute Jembrana disease is characterized by a severe disorder of the lymphoid organs such as the spleen and lymph nodes. If animals survive, they recover completely in one to three months.

The Jembrana disease virus and HIV are actually of the same family: the former is a bovine lentivirus, whereas HIV is a human lentivirus. This is not to say humans acquired HIV or AIDS from cattle. The point is that an HIV-like virus can cause acute and often fatal disease from which some victims recover without recurrence.

In any case, we must seriously question the widespread notion that today's HIV-1B epidemic arose in the United States, without warning, in the 1980s. It now seems that this Western HIV arose in Europe, with several unheeded warnings, as early as 1939. Certainly some form of the agent was causing sporadic cases in Europe—plus at least one small epidemic among newborns—before launching the major epidemic now seen in Europe and the United States. In the 1960s and 1970s, probably due to increased opportunity for passage and circulation, the virus apparently changed from a Jembrana-like human virus to the more lethal HIV we know. It changed from a virus from which recovery is possible to one from which recovery is virtually never possible.

This change may not have required much time. As detailed later, rapid passaging through groups of Asian monkeys changed SIV in only six passages. It started as a virus causing disease in low frequency after a long period of infection. It emerged as a high-frequency and very speedy killer.

3

HIV Baby Booms: Epidemics Rise and Fall

Despite the confusion of Bru and Lai strains, the 1983 and 1984 work of Montagnier and Gallo produced desperately needed antibody tests to diagnose HIV infection and monitor blood supplies. In the United States and Europe, the tests performed quite well. In Africa, however, they seemed to give false-negative results: they did not detect the expected antibodies in patients who clearly had AIDS. For a year or two, this puzzle caused three rumors to circulate. Some researchers said the tests were simply no good. Some said that AIDS was not caused by HIV after all. Others argued that AIDS was indeed caused by HIV but also by other viruses. This last rumor proved closest to the truth.

In 1985 Montagnier and Clavel studied a patient from Guinea-Bissau who definitely had AIDS but no HIV antibodies according to available tests. They found in his blood another virus that seemed in many ways related to Western HIV but different enough to be considered a second AIDS virus. It was named HIV-2, and the original HIV was renamed HIV-1 from then on. HIV-2 was subsequently found in all AIDS cases seronegative for HIV-1, that is, virtually all cases seen in West Africa.

This was the first evidence that AIDS epidemics could spring from different but related virus types. Since that time it has become increasingly clear that worldwide AIDS cannot be explained by a single virus causing a single and continuous epidemic. Instead, worldwide spread is the work of a virus family of types, subtypes, and strains that cause more or less related epidemics. Each member of the family has its own distinctive behavior, and each epidemic runs its own distinctive course.

Now that we have the laboratory tools to identify them, we can look back on the discovery of three HIV types and behaviors: HIV-1 in 1983, HIV-2 in 1985, and HIV-0 in 1990. They are responsible for at least three distinct AIDS epidemics that affect distinct regions of the world. The HIV-1 epidemic spreads rapidly from widely scattered foci; HIV-2 spreads slowly in West Africa and, recently, more rapidly in India; HIV-0 spreads, just barely, in only one part of Africa. These three viruses differ in their appearance, method of transmission, activity, and time and place of occurrence.

To trace the movements and virulence of a particular virus, one must be able to recognize that virus with absolute certainty. A nonvisual method is needed because ordinary microscopy sees cells but not viruses. Electron microscopy sees viruses within cells but is unable to recognize and distinguish HIV types. In 1986 a nonvisual method was discovered by three independent research groups. Two worked in the United States, headed, respectively, by Palker of Duke University and Rusche of Repligen, and one worked in the Netherlands (Meloen and Goudsmit). The method is based on a variable signature site in the outer coat of HIV. Whether type 0, 1, or 2, every HIV contains this site. In its variation, this signature serves to identify not only the HIV type but its subtype and strain.

Similarly, our written signature provides at least three levels of identification. Its script (Arabic, Cyrillic, Latin) places us in a broad cultural group that is analogous to the viral type. Its language (Dutch, French, English) narrows that group to a particular country or ethnic group, analogous to the viral subtype. Finally, the name we write identifies our family, analogous to a viral strain.

What exactly is this viral signature that tells us so much? How is it detected?

As seen in Figure 3.1, HIV has three wrappings. Its shell, or capsid, is surrounded by a membrane (a lipid bilayer, discussed later) plus an envelope. The envelope is not a continuous barrier but a network of two inter-

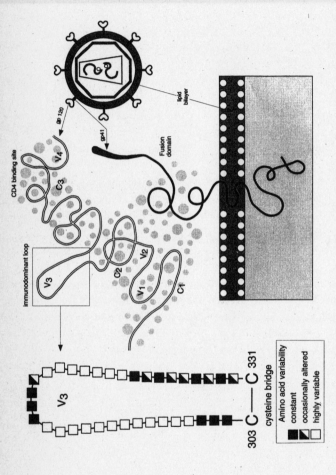

Figure 3.1 **Third variable region (V3) of the HIV-1 envelope protein.** *Of the two envelope proteins, gp41 is rooted in the bilayer membrane and surmounted by gp120, which is loosely connected. This outer molecule includes constant regions (C1, 2, 3) as well as variable regions (V1, 2, 3, 4). The variable regions face outward, toward the target cells. As indicated, some amino acids of the V3 region are constant, some are occasionally altered, and others are highly variable.* (Goudsmit et al., 1988.)

locked proteins that protrude from the membrane much as hairs protrude from our skin. Like all proteins, these envelope proteins consist of amino acids in a particular sequence. In the outermost protein, most of the sequence is fixed, or constant, but a few regions or domains are variable. The so-called third variable domain, or V3, contains the signature site (Figure 3.1). It is a site to which HIV antibodies respond. When we generate antibodies against invaders of our system, they are keyed to very specific parts of those invaders: to certain proteins or, more accurately, to six to ten amino acids within those proteins. The antibodies are configured to bind to this site. When we detect antibody configuration, we learn the topography of their binding site. So when we analyze antibodies to the V3 region of a particular HIV, we detect the topography or signature of that site. This tells us the HIV type, subtype, and strain.

Just one fingerprick of blood from an HIV-infected person (about 10 microliters, or 1/100 of a milliliter) contains one to ten thousand viral particles, which is more than enough for two different methods of signature detection. Antibody analysis, just described, is quick and easy and quite accurate as to virus type. However, it is somewhat less accurate as to subtype and much less accurate as to strain. So for highest accuracy, virologists use molecular techniques to decipher the nucleic acid coding region for the viral signature, that is, the stretch of nucleic acids that codes for the amino acids at the signature site. For HIV this gene fragment can be found in the DNA of host blood cells at points where HIV has been integrated. Alternatively, it can be found in the cell-free HIV RNA that circulates in the host serum.

The molecular method currently requires twenty-four hours for computerized determination and analysis of the viral signature. The result reliably tells you HIV type 0, 1, or 2 and, just as reliably, the subtype and strain. The computer groups viruses by comparing their coding regions and counting the nucleotides by which they differ. In a stretch of about three hundred nucleotides, the HIV types differ by about 40 percent of the nucleotides. Subtypes differ by 20 to 30 percent, and strains by approximately 10 percent. Variants within strains differ by 5 percent. By this same nucleotide yardstick, HIVs and SIVs differ about 60 percent from all other retroviruses. As discussed in Chapter 9, the others are chiefly the lentiviruses of cows, ungulates, and cats; the oncogenic, or cancer-causing, tumor viruses; and the spuma, or "foamy" viruses.

The quick and easy antibody method is usually sufficient for rough distinctions of type and subtype that reveal broad epidemic patterns. It is used to tell whether HIV-0 or HIV-2 is on the move; whether HIV-1 subtype B or E is spreading in Asia; whether HIV-1B is rising or falling in a particular area or moving from one group to another; whether HIV-1C has traveled from Africa to India. However, only the delicate molecular techniques can reliably reveal viral strains. These can tell us who infected whom (e.g., did a Florida dentist infect his patients?) and whether Gallo's HIV-1 IIIB is—or is not—the same as Montagnier's HIV-1 Lai.

Both of these techniques to detect HIV signatures have vastly improved understanding of the current AIDS epidemics. We now know of two virus types, HIV-0 and HIV-2, that cause AIDS in a relatively limited number of people. We know that HIV-2 spreads slowly. We know that both types have been among humans for decades without taking off and causing raging epidemics. HIV-0 has apparently not had the opportunity, but HIV-2 is now spreading in India, suggesting that all types of HIV can spread if given the right opportunity.

Clearly, these HIVs are not harmless to the humans they infect. They are eventually lethal but allow a relatively long symptom-free period compared with HIV-1. They maintain a low level of endemicity in limited parts of the world that are probably close to their animal source or reservoir. In this reservoir they remain a harmless cousin of HIV (i.e., SIV), which may help to explain why they are not more lethal in humans. They have not yet had to change much to adapt to their new host. If allowed to spread rapidly in an environment that is new and far from their reservoir, HIV-0 and HIV-2 might well begin to kill us more quickly.

More about Viral Sex

HIV-2 has at least three subtypes (maybe many more), none of which is confined to just one geographic area. HIV-2 subtype A is found in Senegal, the Cape Verde Islands, Mali, Ghana, Gambia, and Guinea-Bissau. HIV-2 subtype B is widespread in West Africa. Nowhere is either subtype a great threat to the general population, but since both HIV-2A and HIV-2B circulate in West Africa, they can infect cells of the same individual. This leads to viral sex and recombinant offspring, as are seen in many cases of West African HIV-2 infection.

We must briefly review the mating habits of HIV because, as mentioned in the preface, they are its secret weapon and potentially ours too. Like humans, HIV has two identical copies of each gene, but we have twenty-three pairs of chromosomes, each pair containing about seventy-five thousand genes. The virus has the equivalent of one pair, which contains ten genes. Our genes are strung along double-stranded DNA within chromosomes. HIV makes do with single-stranded RNA and no chromosomal packaging. Paradoxically for such a small and genetically deprived creature, HIV reproduction is more complex than human reproduction in two important respects.

First, HIV reproduction requires the active participation of a third party: the living host cell. HIV can enter and infect its favorite immune cell at any time, but the virus is quiescent as long as the cell is quiescent. It cannot do its damage until converted to DNA and integrated into the cell genome. This happens when the resting cell is activated by the threat of some foreign invader. When the immune cell multiplies in response to the invader, HIV enters the cell genome and begins to multiply, using the cellular reproductive machinery.

Second, whereas most organisms have only one reproductive choice, HIVs have two choices. They can reproduce sexually, by the mating of two parents (our only choice), or they can reproduce asexually (the only choice of most microorganisms). In asexual reproduction, the genes of one generation are copied or cloned to the next. Sexual reproduction can also produce clones, as when a host cell is infected by two identical viruses, that is, HIVs having two identical strands of RNA. By definition, clones are exact copies, but HIV cloning is careless and produces many inexact copies. This accounts for some of the change we see in the HIV family, though not the remarkable pace or degree of change. It does not explain the successive new waves of HIV that are quite distinct from their parents yet still able to cause AIDS.

Such change is possible only with sexual reproduction and recombination (see Figure I.1). This requires infection of the host cell by viruses that are not identical but have enough genetic overlap to permit crossover of genetic information. Their mating produces offspring of three kinds. Two are homozygous, that is, one has two identical RNA strands like one parent;

the other has two identical RNA strands like the other parent. The third is heterozygous, having one RNA strand from each parent. These heterozygotes look like either parent but have characteristics of both. They do not, themselves, represent remarkable change, but their mating does. When heterozygotes infect a new cell, they produce recombinant offspring. Each virus of this new generation has two identical RNA strands that mix genes of both father and mother.

Recombinant offspring are not always better than their parents, but recombination allows variation and flexibility. In retroviruses like HIV that reproduce quickly and often, recombination allows major change in a short time. It can eliminate mutations from the father or mother that are deleterious to the virus. It can enable rapid adaptation to a new host or mode of transmission. HIVs continually mate and produce recombinant offspring—completely new viruses with completely new characteristics—which predicts that AIDS epidemics will continually rise and fall around the world.

A Global Survey of HIV

The many recombinant offspring of HIV-2A and HIV-2B tell us that these two subtypes have long inhabited the same region and population, causing double infections in many individuals. Their confinement, until recently, to very restricted and overlapping areas in West Africa suggests a local source for HIV-2. It could be human or some nonhuman primate, as discussed in Chapter 6.

Only in West Africa are there regions where the majority of AIDS cases are caused by HIV-2. Even in regions where HIV-1 now has the lion's share, HIV-2 keeps a small but steady percentage of all HIV infections. However, its share of AIDS cases is even smaller than its share of HIV infections. Since HIV-2 infections progress to AIDS very slowly or not at all, the great majority (over 95 percent) of AIDS in West Africa is caused by HIV-1, largely subtype A.

Exposure to HIV-2 leads much less frequently to infection and AIDS than does exposure to HIV-1A. Recent evidence suggests that individuals exposed to both HIV-2 and HIV-1A may gain some benefit from HIV-2. It does not completely protect against infection by HIV-1A, since many individuals show evidence of both infections. But it may slow the rapid disease course of HIV-1A since HIV-2 infects the same type of cell as HIV-1. The fact that they are cross-competitors suggests that these viruses are related and evolved from a distant common ancestor. If so, HIV-1 has evolved much farther from the presumably harmless ancestor because it is now far more harmful than HIV-2.

Both HIV-2 and HIV-1A are typically transmitted by heterosexual (i.e., vaginal) intercourse, but HIV-2 seems ill adapted to this route. It rarely establishes a new infection and when it does, the infection is low-grade, resulting in a slow and sometimes inapparent disease course. In a low-grade infection, diagnosis is possible but isolation of the virus is difficult. The HIV-2 virus load is small and causes only short periods of acute illness. Individuals infected with HIV-2 rarely develop AIDS.

This picture of low infectivity and slow disease course will probably remain as long as the opportunity to transmit HIV-2 remains low. The opportunity is unlikely to change in West Africa and, when HIV-2 appears in Europe and Asia, it so far appears in West African immigrants or their partners. If HIV-2 remains thus limited to its accustomed place and people, it may never take off. But the history of HIV-1 warns against complacency.

The vast majority of people infected with HIV-2 show a disease course like that seen in a tiny minority of those infected with HIV-1, the so-called nonprogressors. Those in this rare group, including our two men in Amsterdam, have very few virus particles circulating in their blood. Most people infected with HIV-1 have many circulating particles, or virions, and the more they have, the more rapidly AIDS develops. We must suspect that any process able to increase the HIV-2 virus load will make it more threatening, perhaps ultimately as threatening as HIV-1.

Such a scenario is not hard to imagine. All it takes is an individual with HIV-2 infection who has an unusually high and persistent virus load. He or she would have the mild but prolonged infectivity to transmit the virus to one or more individuals, especially if they engaged in activities like frequent unprotected anal sex. Since HIV-2 spreads poorly by heterosexual relations, it may spread better by homosexual relations. If so, one fears that HIV-2 is potentially as dangerous as HIV-1. It simply has not yet bumped into the population that can spread it rapidly. We have seen that rapid circulation alone can start a chain reaction of HIV infections that progress faster and more frequently to AIDS. If HIV-2A is now spreading heterosexually among prostitutes in India, this scenario may already be under way.

The story of HIV-0 is in many respects very similar to the story of HIV-2. In 1990, in a couple from Cameroon, van der Groen and Piot found HIV strains highly divergent from HIV-1 and HIV-2. Several other research teams subsequently isolated similar strains from other AIDS patients, all from Cameroon or Gabon. Many of these patients showed no HIV-1 or HIV-2 antibodies in response to the customary HIV tests. They were infected with strains now designated HIV-0, which infects almost exclusively people living in Cameroon and Gabon. The virus has been found in Europe but, as with HIV-2, it has been found only in immigrants from its source countries or in their sex partners. Even in Cameroon and Gabon, HIV-0 infections are extremely rare. Among HIV-positive individuals in those areas, the culprit is usually HIV-1A, and this is even more the case among those who have AIDS. The situation echoes HIV-2 versus HIV-1A in West Africa.

At this point about twenty HIV-0 strains have been isolated. Study of their signature V3 sequences suggests that this virus is at least as variable as HIV-1. But whereas HIV-1 subtypes tend to have diverse habitats, HIV-0 strains share the same or overlapping habitats. Their distinguishing features are as yet unclear, either because data are lacking or because their differentiation is incomplete. As will be discussed toward the end of this chapter, distinct HIV subtypes are believed to form through competition and adaptation to various hosts. HIV-0 lacks subtypes because it has not yet faced these challenges.

HIV-0 infections have so far occurred only after heterosexual transmission. They are far less widespread than infections with HIV-1A or any other heterosexually transmitted HIV-1 subtypes. But as with HIV-2, this does not mean HIV-0 could not become a killer under the right circumstances. At this point, we may see HIV-0 and HIV-2 stalled or suspended at a stage that HIV-1 left decades ago. HIV-1 has moved on and now rarely behaves like HIV-2. For HIV-2, the picture is reversed: it rarely behaves like the more virulent HIV-1. Sparse data on HIV-0 keep us guessing about its strength. However, like HIV-2, it has not reached high infectivity and therefore, though ultimately fatal, it does not threaten to become stronger and more widespread in its home area. Both HIV-2 and HIV-0 remain confined and unrelated to the mainstream AIDS epidemic, but they could soar, given the chance.

Clearly AIDS can be caused by more than one HIV type, though HIV-1 is currently the main killer. Figure 3.2 shows that HIV-1B dominates in Europe and the United States, while HIV-1A is more common in Africa. Are

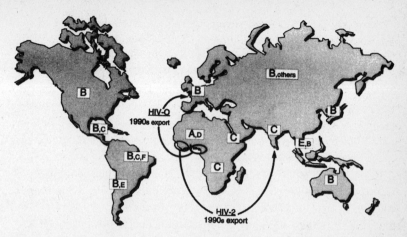

Figure 3.2   Global distribution of HIV-1 types and subtypes in the 1990s.
*HIV-0, HIV-1, and HIV-2 are found in Africa. HIV-2 has been exported to India
and HIV-0 to Europe, but neither has yet caused a major epidemic. HIV-1B,
agent of the Western AIDS epidemic, still dominates Europe and the Americas,
although HIV-1C is rising in South America. HIV-1B also dominates Eastern
Europe (along with other subtypes), as well as Japan and Australia. In Southeast
Asia, HIV-1E is rising fast, along with C. In Africa, HIV-1A dominates, along
with C. The distribution suggests that subtypes spread mainly by heterosexual
transmission (Asia, Africa) tend to outcompete subtypes spread mainly by homosexual transmission (Europe, the Americas), and vice versa. One group tends to
dominate and even exclude the other in a given population niche. (Lukashov,
Kuiken and Goudsmit, 1995.)*

these the only HIV-1 subtypes? Are they the same or similar in their level of
infectivity, virulence, and mode of transmission?

As might be expected from our comparison of HIV-0, HIV-1, and HIV-2,
the answer is a resounding no. Eight subtypes of HIV-1 have already been
identified. Labeled A through H, they show remarkable geographic separation, in contrast to the overlapping strains and subtypes of HIV-0 and HIV-2.
Apparently, once a HIV-1 subtype is established in a geographic niche,
other HIV-1 subtypes have difficulty penetrating that area. This is the net
effect of what may be considered a viral war. Multiple HIV-1 subtypes may
move into a certain population, but depending on their infectivity or transmission characteristics, one subtype will pull ahead in the competition. It
survives and wins the niche because, by definition, it is the fittest: it

spreads most efficiently in the population. More rarely, two or more subtypes with equal advantages will end up sharing a population.

However, win or draw, the viral war goes on. Peace is only temporary because stronger and more aggressive subtypes keep turning up. No matter how
perfectly subtypes are adapted to their hosts, they can always be displaced by
changes in the population (e.g., in sexual practices) or changes in competing
subtypes. At any moment, the formerly fittest subtype can be overtaken by
one even more fit. A niche holder may lose its hold, especially if recombination suddenly produces a subtype with markedly superior advantages.

These notions point to subtype-specific AIDS epidemics that are separate and distinct in time, location, and other features. Their agents are separate and distinct in transmission route, infectivity, and aggressivity. They
do not merge despite continual strain variation within subtypes. Since the
beginning of the AIDS epidemic in Amsterdam, we have studied more than
a hundred HIV-1B strains in newly infected individuals. What we observed
was quite remarkable. As expected, strain variation (as indicated by the V3
signature site) accumulated as the epidemic progressed and involved more
individuals. However, over these ten to twelve years of viral replication, the
strains remained recognizable as members of subtype B. They infected
thousands of new hosts and went through millions of replication cycles.
Each replication yielded mutation of at least one of the 10,000 nucleic
acids of the AIDS virus genome. But the virus infecting people in 1990
looked surprisingly similar to the virus infecting people in 1980.

This stability strongly suggests that early in an epidemic, a particular
AIDS virus adapts rapidly to its host. It evolves optimal reproduction characteristics for a particular method of virus dissemination. Subsequently, all
strains of the virus population conserve the genetic characteristics that
have guaranteed the success of their subtype. That is, the strains with
these characteristics thrive while those without them disappear.

Some HIV-1 subtypes occupy very large territories; others rule small
areas. There is good reason to believe that, whatever their realm, the subtype-specific epidemics are prone to change at any time. A subtype can
even die out, if only because its most infectious strains die with their victims. In fact, we see evidence that the HIV-1B epidemic has peaked in the
West. In the United States and Europe, it seems to be fading, at least from
its primary risk groups of gay men and IV drug users. The number of new
HIV-1B infections in these groups has stopped rising and may even be declining, especially in Western Europe. It looks as if the first major HIV-1B

epidemic has completed its natural cycle of logarithmic increase and has begun its retreat.

As discussed earlier, HIV-1B may well have been endemic in Europe long before the American outbreak of the early 1980s. With a low level of infectivity and aggressivity, it resembled today's HIV-2 (lethal but slow) or the Jembrana virus of cattle (not always lethal). It rarely caused disease following heterosexual transmission or blood transmission. However, once it entered the emancipated gay community, it adapted to invade humans through the inner walls of the rectum. Rapid circulation allowed it to become the efficient killer we see today. In the United States, for the first ten to fifteen years of the epidemic, about 50 percent of all AIDS cases occurred among gay men. In Europe the percentage was smaller, but only because it combined the very low percentage of gay AIDS cases in southern Europe (where AIDS is seen mainly in IV drug users) with the very high percent in northern Europe. In northern cities like Amsterdam, 75 percent of AIDS cases still occur in the gay community.

In general, HIV-1B may be fading slightly among gay men and IV drug users, but this does not mean that AIDS will vanish from the Western world. Subtypes could be imported that excel HIV-1B in their rate of heterosexual transmission. Studies in Thailand show that HIV-1E has a 75 percent chance of heterosexual transmission, whereas HIV-1B has a 25 percent chance. In other words, of one hundred people exposed to HIV-1E by heterosexual relations, seventy-five are likely to be infected; with HIV-1B, twenty-five are likely to be infected. For HIV-1B to cause a heterosexual epidemic, a homosexual or anal factor seems to be required. In Haiti, for example, HIV was probably introduced by gay tourists from the United States who sought sex with young male prostitutes. The Haitian men they infected with HIV-1B then infected wives and girlfriends, particularly since heterosexual couples in Latin America commonly use anal sex as a "no-cost" contraceptive measure.

In most of the United States and Western Europe, other contraceptive measures are generally affordable and preferred. For this and other cultural reasons, anal sex is less popular among heterosexual couples in these regions, so their risk of HIV-1B infection remains relatively low. But if not displaced by a more efficient subtype, HIV-1B could change. It could come to rely less on anal transmission and more on vaginal transmission. Some data suggest that because certain cells (e.g., Langerhans' cells) are more abundant in vaginal than rectal tissue, the HIVs best at vaginal transmission are those best at entering these cells. HIV-1B strains with this knack could someday appear and gradually outcompete HIV-1B strains limited to anal transmission. As always, this would be a random process, not the result of a viral conspiracy! Natural selection simply favors the preservation and accumulation of *accidental* changes that prove to be advantageous. In this case, strains with the knack would simply survive better than those without it.

A fierce debate rages as to whether HIV-1B has already begun to change. There is strong concern that it is shifting from the population of gay men and IV drug users to the general population, especially women. The percentage of US women among AIDS patients has indeed risen since 1985—even doubled, according to some data. However, a similar rise has not been seen in Europe, and we lack hard evidence that HIV-1B has actually become more efficient in spreading to women. Three factors help to explain this apparent contradiction.

First of all, as gay men decrease their share of total AIDS cases, women's share increases even if their actual number of cases remains the same. Second, some US women who are counted as AIDS patients have HIV infection combined with female diseases like cervical cancer. These diseases or their treatment can aggravate HIV infection and hasten development of AIDS. They do not themselves cause immunodeficiency but, since 1993, women with such diseases have been defined as AIDS patients when HIV infection is also present. Finally, if HIV-1B actually infects more US women, they are primarily women of a certain behavioral group, not women in general. They are poor black and Hispanic women of US inner cities, but their AIDS risk is only marginally tied to poverty, race, or sex with an HIV-positive partner. It is mainly tied to drug use. In New York, for example, two-thirds of the black and Hispanic women with AIDS are IV drug users. Of the rest, most have sex with a drug user. If a poor black or Hispanic woman lives in a community at high risk for AIDS *but avoids drug use and sex with drug users*, her chance of infection is negligible. It thus appears that HIV-1B has not actually or appreciably improved its rate of heterosexual transmission.

Of course, the virus is bound to move from the gay to the general population, especially in urban centers. How much and how fast this happens varies from city to city depending, in each locale, on the distance and interface between the gay population and the drug-using population of the inner city. Still, heterosexual transmission per se seems to have little impact on the inner-city spread of HIV. Except among IV drug users, such transmission remains rare unless assisted by special circumstances: preexisting venereal disease, or unusually high virus load in the male partner, or anal intercourse. Studies in Thailand showed that even frequency of intercourse did not promote the transmission of HIV-1B as long as the intercourse was vaginal, not anal.

Thailand is the main focus of HIV-1 B in Southeast Asia. The virus has also been exported to South America, mainly Brazil. In Thailand it first surfaced in 1987 among IV drug users in the southern capital city of Bangkok. So HIV-1 subtype B had apparently spread from Europe to the United States and Haiti, then to Thailand. It is not far-fetched to assume that its spread was related to sex tourism followed by dissemination in the Thai IV drug–using population. Thailand may have no more prostitution than other Asian countries, but its commercial sex industry is more socially and officially accepted. Younger and younger women are working as prostitutes because they can be promoted as virgins, free of HIV. They are often recruited from remote villages to ensure minimal exposure to sex or disease. A convenient myth circulates that young girls, even nonvirgins, are somehow impervious to HIV. To its credit, Thailand has now begun to work hard on HIV-related problems.

In 1989 a second HIV-1 epidemic emerged in the north of Thailand, but the agent was subtype E. Rarely seen before, HIV-1E rapidly spread south by heterosexual transmission, invading the territory of subtype B: the IV drug users. Today subtype B is becoming scarce throughout Thailand and is not spreading to the rest of Asia. This again proves that HIV-1B is well adapted to spread and do harm through anal sexual intercourse but ill adapted to do harm through vaginal intercourse. It competes poorly with subtypes more efficient in heterosexual transmission.

In West Africa and other parts of Africa, HIV-1A is the dominant AIDS-causing virus. Spread easily through heterosexual intercourse, it is overtaking the slow but steady HIV-2 and is competing with HIV-1D for dominance in central Africa. Whether 1A or 1D will win is unclear. Already we see recombinants of A and D viruses, so the victory may go to descendants with the best characteristics of both. Wherever they occur, recombination events sustain HIV and AIDS by adding new viruses to the circulating mix. Recently, a study of Rwandan women documented the emergence of an

HIV-1A/C recombinant that is already capable of infection and transmission to a new host.

HIV-1A has not spread to Asia, but its genes have. The emerging threat to Asians, HIV-1E, is actually a recombinant virus that inherited all its genes from HIV-1A, except the one that codes for the viral envelope. That gene comes from its other parent. The recombination event probably occurred in central Africa since both HIV-1A and the recombinant 1E are found there. Remarkably, the parent that contributed the envelope gene has not yet been found anywhere. It is very rare or even extinct, suggesting that the recombination event must have occurred long ago.

The fact that HIV-1E spreads much better in Asia than in Africa points strongly to host or genetic factors. Apparently, the cells of Asians are more susceptible to 1E infection than to 1A infection and, conversely, the cells of Africans are more susceptible to 1A than 1E. The theory is that central African drug smugglers, infected with HIV-1E, brought the virus to Thailand. The virus is so infectious through heterosexual intercourse that it is now spreading in all of Asia with devastating effects. In its rapid journey through Asia, it has learned to spread very fast in a dense population. If we could stop only one AIDS virus, it should be this one, since it threatens by far the largest concentration of people (Figure 3.3).

As far as we know, the only other AIDS virus now on the rise is HIV-1 subtype C. This virus was first documented among the populations of Ethiopia and Somalia. It then moved south to South Africa and its neighbors, and from there to India by a path similar to that followed by HIV-2A. HIV-1C recently emerged in Central America and has also reached China.

In the spread of various subtypes, China is an important and special case. At first, all reported cases were HIV-1B. They occurred in Yunnan Province, which has points of contact with Vietnam, Laos, Thailand, and Myanmar (Burma). But the virus was actually a Thai variant, known as HIV-1B', which probably entered China with infected drug users or dealers crossing the Yunnan border. At the same time, Chinese women who had worked in Thailand as prostitutes came back infected with HIV-1E. But since 1990, most strains found among infected drug users of Yunnan are HIV-1C. Not found in Thailand, this subtype has apparently come to China from some other area, so far unknown. A viral war between subtypes C and E seems imminent in this part of the world.

So we see that AIDS is not caused by a single virus but by very different viruses from one big HIV family. Each one of the family can cause AIDS

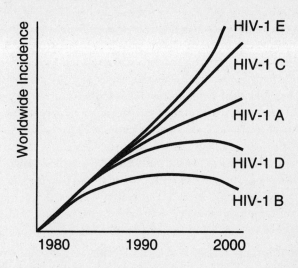

Figure 3.3 **Worldwide incidence and shift of HIV-1 subtypes.** *Since 1980, the focus of worldwide AIDS has shifted from HIV-1B in Europe and the Americas to HIV-1E and C in Asia. As of 1995, E and C are rising the fastest, and B is declining or leveling off. (D also has declined but was never widespread.) HIV-1A is still strong and rising but is outstripped by the Asian subtypes because they dominate denser populations.*

but at various rates—an important distinguishing feature. Some have acquired the characteristic to be infectious primarily through entry in the gut of men and women (i.e., the anal mucosa of the lower intestine), while others are more infectious through entry in the vagina (or the penis, though this is relatively rare). Some of these viruses, like HIV-0 and HIV-2, are endemic in very small regions of the world. They have not yet caused large-scale AIDS epidemics, mainly because they have not encountered the right opportunity. HIV-1B had the opportunity and caused a large epidemic that now seems to be winding down. Meanwhile, others are on the rise, threatening epidemics of immense proportions: HIV-1E and C in Asia; HIV-1A and D in Africa.

We see no indication that HIV-1 subtypes are merging into one super-subtype. And in the course of an epidemic, though variation accumulates within the responsible subtype, every new strain looks very much like those that infected people at the beginning of that epidemic. However, we see that one subtype can overtake another, as is now happening in Thailand.

When a subtype is battling another for dominance, the losing virus has only one chance for survival. It can pass its genes to the conquering virus through recombination. Viruses of the HIV family continually interbreed to perpetuate the family trade, even at the cost of an individual virus subtype or strain. Viral sex allows variation while preserving the unique genetic characteristics of the family: the ability to replicate and spread through cells of the immune system of the host. All members of the family infect a host by entering CD4+ immune cells, where they replicate. The offspring burst from the cells into extracellular fluid, by which they are transmitted (by sexual relations or exchange of blood) to a new host and breeding ground. Or, before they burst out, the virus particles are transmitted within the infected cell and are disgorged in the new host. Either way, the old host is then useless, and the parent viruses are headed for extinction. Their fate does not matter, now that the offspring have found a new host. However, the moribund parent viruses continue to circulate, eventually causing AIDS and killing the discarded host.

HIV types and subtypes can be considered distinct viruses since they remain stable while accommodating enormous strain variation. Even if they share a common ancestor, their distribution history will vary, depending on many circumstances. As an example, we can look at the history of HIV-1B in Thailand. The virus surfaced in 1987 and within a year had started an AIDS epidemic among IV drug users in Bangkok. In one to two years, it was spreading from IV drug users to male and female prostitutes and their clients, particularly soldiers. The virus circulating among IV drug users seemed to be the same virus circulating sexually, but this was not quite true. By the early 1990s, the virus of Bangkok drug users belonged to the HIV-1B subtype and probably came from the West. However, a close look found genetic differences that put it in a new category. Now called HIV-1B', it is similar to HIV-1B but very distinct from HIV-1E, the sub-group spreading rapidly in Thailand and the rest of Asia. Initially, the E virus was found largely in cases of sexual transmission, not transmission by drug use. HIV-1E infected very few IV drug users in the late 1980s but is now overtaking both HIV-1B and HIV-1B' in that risk group. By the time this book is published, we expect 1B and 1B' to have virtually disappeared from Thailand.

Researchers at the Centers for Disease Control in Atlanta have recently traced the history of HIV-1B, HIV-1B', and HIV-1E in Thailand, mainly by looking at two groups of Thai prison inmates. The first group included ten drug users infected with HIV-1B in 1986 and 1987, before the Thai epidemic took off. The second included three men who were infected once the epidemic was in full swing: one by HIV-1E and two by HIV-1B'. In the first group the ten infecting strains were indistinguishable from those circulating in Europe and the United States. They were true HIV-1 subtype B, and even had the same signature in the V3 region as Euro-American strains, which strongly suggests that they were imported by Euro-American travelers. The ten early-infected men left prison in 1988. They were then free to spread HIV-1B in the drug-using community, but the virus did not thrive. In the West it had been passaged to greater virulence by homosexual intercourse before it entered the drug-using population. This did not happen in Thailand to any great extent. In the West it had no competitors, but in Thailand it faced HIV-1E and HIV-1B'. After 1988, HIV-1B was edged out by HIV-1B' among drug users, while HIV-1 subtype E spread simultaneously among prostitutes through heterosexual intercourse. Now HIV-1B' is also fading from drug users, edged out by HIV-1E. Clearly, a given HIV virus can be readily replaced—in only a few years—by an HIV better suited for spread in a particular population.

A population may be defined by many factors, ranging from behavior to racial or ethnic group. Just as HIV-1B and HIV-1B' are less successful than HIV-1E in a heterosexual population, they may also be less successful among certain Asian peoples. As individuals worldwide vary in their strengths and weaknesses—including their susceptibility to this or that disease—so do ethnic groups. They are, after all, collections of individuals who share a common background and physiology, however diluted by time and distance. All other things being equal, host factors make a difference. Many diseases vary in prevalence from Caucasians to Africans to Asians. Many occur in just one subgroup that has special susceptibility. For example, Tay-Sachs disease occurs almost exclusively among northeast European Jews or their descendants, regardless of where those descendants live today. The rarity of HIV-1B among Africans suggests that they resist it better than do Euro-Americans. Perhaps Asians also resist HIV-1B while being, like Africans, easy prey to other subtypes.

The Outgrowth of Subtypes

If one HIV-1 subtype can quickly overtake and replace another, the question is, Are they truly different viruses with different distribution histories, or are they essentially one virus that has rapidly formed subgroups in adapting to various risk groups? A related question is, Do HIV-1 subtypes predate the AIDS outbreak of the early 1980s, or have they developed in these past fifteen years?

If they are truly different viruses, their worldwide spread is directed by chance within transmissibility limits, since subtypes are not equally well spread by anal or vaginal intercourse. This seems indicated by a small study we performed in Russia, Byelorussia, and Lithuania. The viruses we studied in the former Soviet Union did not cluster geographically but according to risk groups based on behavior. Thus, of seven HIV-infected people who had acquired the virus by homosexual intercourse, all seven were infected by HIV-1B, whether they lived in Vilnius, Lithuania, or Moscow. Of six heterosexually infected people, all six had HIV-1C, whether residents of Minsk, Byelorussia, or Rostov in Russia. Perhaps most ominous, four people infected through drug use in various cities had four different types: HIV-1A, C, D, and G. Apparently, any subtype passes with ease among drug users, whether it is suited to anal or vaginal transmission. If so, IV drug use is the best and perhaps the main vehicle for a subtype to enter a new area. However, once introduced, a new subtype may fail to thrive, as HIV-1B has so far failed in Thailand.

That the HIV-1 subtypes were truly separate well before the 1980s can be extrapolated from the genetic history of HIV-1A and 1B, the two we know best. HIV-1A was first isolated from a sample taken in Tanzania in 1976. Allowing for strain variation, that virus is indistinguishable from today's HIV-1A viruses, so the origin of the subtypes must lie before 1976 and, more specifically, before the AIDS epidemic became apparent. Subtype emergence most likely resulted from the successful adaptation of HIV to spread in the human population. The same can be said for HIV-1B. The viruses isolated from individuals infected in Amsterdam in the early 1980s are not markedly different from those found in people infected ten years later. And if one believes the history related in Chapter 2, HIV-1B has been stable for more than forty years.

The genetic data on HIV-1A and 1B indicate that neither is the ancestor of the other. Also, HIV-1 subtypes are relatively stable on a gene-by-gene basis. Point mutations of genes result in proliferation of strains within a subtype, but strains do not leave the subtype or merge with other strains. Some subtypes show more strain variation than others, so either their evolution is faster or they are older. In any case, subtypes must be independent entities that predate the epidemic status of HIV (though not necessarily its ability to cause immune deficiency). For at least two decades— millions of generations for HIV—the subtypes have been genetically stable entities in which point mutations can occur without loss of basic characteristics defining the subtype.

If the HIV-0, HIV-1, and HIV-2 types and subtypes predate any AIDS epidemic, where did they originate? As to HIV-0 and HIV-2, the answer is relatively easy. They have so far caused only small outbreaks of AIDS in Africa. Their appearance on other continents has been traced directly back to Africa. So they originated in Africa.

The same is less clear-cut but appears to be true for the HIV-1 subtypes. All those known to us can be found somewhere in Africa even if, like HIV-1B, they are very rare on that continent. More important, multiple HIV-1 subtypes have cocirculated in several parts of Africa and, until very recently, on no other continent. Since cocirculation of subtypes is necessary for creation of new subtypes, Africa was the first place this process could occur, as far as we know.

As explained, new subtypes result when two nonidentical parent subtypes infect a single host cell. If they produce a recombinant virus particularly fit for survival in a particular population, it may become a viable new—and even dominant—subtype, such as HIV-1E in Asia. The chance for such success depends on the level at which subtypes cocirculate, and on the frequency of new infections. As one or both rise, the resulting rise in recombinants—in sheer number and genetic variety—increases the potential for new subtypes.

About 10 percent of worldwide HIV-1 viruses can be earmarked as recombinants of HIV-1 subtypes. All HIV-1 subtypes have participated in recombination, as have all HIV-2 subtypes. But HIV-1 and HIV-2 subtypes mix only among themselves, not with each other. HIV-1 subtypes are sexually incompatible with HIV-2 subtypes. Like humans and chimpanzees, they are closely related but cannot mate and produce a hybrid. Whether HIV-0 viruses can mate and produce recombinants with HIV-1 or HIV-2 viruses is unlikely and so far not described despite the recent description of individuals coinfected with HIV-0 and HIV-1. That is the main reason I use the term HIV-0, unlike those researchers who group HIV-0 viruses with HIV-1 as "subtype O" (see Chapter 5). I may be shown wrong, if and when wider circulation of HIV-0 in HIV-1 and HIV-2 endemic areas produces recombinant offspring.

So the birth of today's many HIV subtypes required, at the beginning, the cocirculation and mating of at least two from each type: HIV-0, HIV-1, and HIV-2. These six parent subtypes must have emerged previously from dramatic events, such as cross-species transmissions, in Africa. After passing from their animal reservoir to humans, these progenitor subtypes pursued their independent ways, adapting to new environments and spawning variants. Such far-reaching development is plausible because their histories span several decades. If AIDS in Europe dates back to the eve of World War II, then the HIV family must go back still farther.

4

The Rain Forest
Roots of HIV-1

The Western AIDS epidemic of the early 1980s was foreshadowed by a subtle epidemic that began in Germany in 1939. With hindsight, we know it spread to other European countries and killed many children, but its pattern and significance were long unnoticed. Its agent was apparently a primitive form of HIV-1B that was not yet strong enough to cause AIDS as we know it. This "proto-1B" caused acute immunodeficiency in most infected people but chronic or fatal disease in very few. Mainly newborns were susceptible, and most recovered with no recurrence. Only later, in the permissive 1960s and 1970s, would proto-1B cycle to greater virulence and become HIV-1B, the inexorable killer of adults.

The virus we are calling proto-1B must have come to Germany from Africa. Since it surfaced on the eve of World War II, was the war a factor in its introduction to Europe? Where did it come from in Africa, and why did it land in Germany? Using scarce data as stepping-stones, we can trace a probable history of HIV-1B and the rest of the HIV-1 family.

HIV-1B is extremely rare in Africa, but a few strains have been found in certain countries of the sub-Saharan rain forest: Gabon, Cameroon, Ivory Coast, Uganda, and Rwanda. Proto-1B must have reached Europe from one of these areas, but probably not Uganda or Rwanda. Before 1940, the lack of commercial air transportation made these interior countries virtually inaccessible. The virus more likely came by ship from a coastal area. It could have come from Ivory Coast, then a French colony, but since the 1939 epidemic began in Germany, a German colony is more logical. This points to Cameroon, which then included the northern parts of Gabon.

Proto-1B must have descended from the African ancestor of all HIV-1 subtypes. Two theories are possible: either this common ancestor evolved in Cameroon, or it evolved elsewhere, and the direct ancestor of proto-1B was subsequently planted in Cameroon. The latter seems unlikely because it implies a degree of evolution that would have made the virus more harmful and noticeable than it apparently was. Even if not always fatal, a serious disease would have been noticed in Cameroon, a colony with a good infrastructure dating back to the nineteenth century. Historical records would tell us if a deadly illness was endemic among colonists or local plantation workers. It would have made the country less prosperous and attractive to European superpowers, but England, France, and Germany never stopped fighting for this treasure. No reports hint that Cameroon was a dangerous place to colonize. So we can assume that, in colonial times, most HIV strains circulating in the territory must have been harmless and unnoticeable. They were largely unable to cause disease and, as will be argued, had not yet grown into subtypes. The strain that became proto-1B had deadly potential but perhaps never caused *P. carinii* pneumonia (PCP) or other opportunistic infections and tumors until it got to Europe. This odd variant that mutated into a disease-causing virus no doubt left Cameroon by sheer chance.

Proto-1B would have been closely related to the common HIV-1 ancestor, so that ancestor must have lived nearby. Whereas proto-1B ultimately went to Europe, other descendant strains traveled eastward in Africa. Like proto-1B, they would evolve from harmless to AIDS-causing viruses, mainly HIV-1A. This would happen in Zaire or Uganda, which saw the first African AIDS cases in the 1970s. The African AIDS epidemic clearly emerged there, just west of Lake Victoria (Figure 4.1). And if HIV subtypes form only during an epidemic in which disease is linked to passage among human hosts, then this same area gave rise to all the HIV-1 subtypes that favor heterosexual transmission. Only HIV-1B, which favors homosexual transmission, developed its full potential elsewhere—in Europe. This historical scenario, with its two paths, may explain the divergence of 1B from

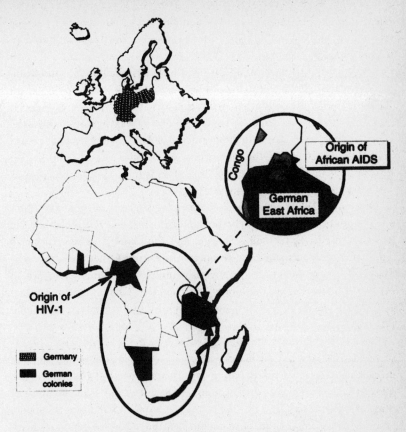

Figure 4.1   Travel of HIV-1 to East Africa. *European or African soldiers, sailors, adventurers, or servants could easily have brought HIV-1 to East Africa at the turn of the century. Hatched areas show German colonies (about 1900), including Cameroon, where HIV-1 was first transmitted from monkey to humans; and German East Africa, where African AIDS emerged near Lake Victoria in the mid-1970s. (McEvedy 1980.)*

the others: its preferential spread through anal intercourse versus their spread through vaginal intercourse.

Since the common ancestor in Cameroon was harmless, a few HIV-1 strains could unknowingly be transported eastward, where they would quietly evolve by heterosexual passage. Likewise, strains that remained in Cameroon and Gabon evolved, unnoticed, into what became proto-1B.

Then, during epidemics in Europe and the United States, they formed HIV-1B, the only HIV-1 subtype formed through serial passage by anal intercourse.

The common ancestor of HIV-1 must have passed from its source animal to humans in some outlying part of Cameroon, in the deep rain forest where people would be hunting and eating this animal. Once cross-species transmission had occurred, a human epidemic was perhaps inevitable. Given enough time, the natural movements of African peoples might eventually have given HIV-1 the opportunity to become a large-scale human killer. But as it happened, the evolution of dangerous HIV-1 subtypes was vastly assisted by German colonialism.

During the 1880s, the African continent was rapidly occupied by European nations, particularly the French and British. The French claimed the tip of West Africa, including Senegal and the Gambia, where they had maintained outposts since the seventeenth century. Other areas taken by the French were new to them: Algeria, Tunisia, and Gabon. The British settled in Sierra Leone, the Gold Coast (modern Ghana), and the Cape, where they had displaced the Dutch in 1806. Egypt was added to the empire in 1882.

Because these powers moved so vigorously to carve up Africa, others moved to take a share. Bismarck laid claim to all areas in which German missionaries were active, including Togo, Cameroon, and German Southwest Africa. Germany claimed Cameroon in July 1884. In December of that year, a representative of the Society of German Colonization signed a treaty with the inhabitants of mainland Zanzibar. This territory later overlapped with British Tanganyika and is now part of Tanzania. In 1887 it became German East Africa, to which the Germans soon added Rwanda and Burundi. Germany kept all these colonies about forty years, until the end of World War I.

European colonialism caused turmoil in Africa, especially the mixing and movement of peoples. Europeans not uncommonly had sexual relations with their subject people. In Cameroon, for example, many German officials reportedly had local black mistresses. These relationships sometimes erupted in scandal and bloodshed. For example, one Lieutenant Schenneman is recorded to have had village men castrated because his black mistress had had affairs with three of them. Even Carl Peters, the founding father of German East Africa, committed such atrocities. A few years after being appointed imperial commissioner in 1891, he illegally hanged his African servant, Mabruk, because of suspected relations with Jagodja, Peters's black mistress. Jagodja was also hanged. Probably such notorious cases were only the tip of the iceberg. Many less notable Germans colonists no doubt had short- or long-term sexual relationships with local people. In any case, we can assume that circulating HIV strains, though relatively harmless, were sometimes passed from Africans to Germans by sexual transmission.

In this same period there were major military movements against subject people who rebelled against cruelty and injustice. Such movements of the army and particularly the navy gave HIV ample opportunity to spread from one territory to another. It is easily envisioned that, around the turn of the century, a German sailor or adventurer—or an African servant—became infected in Cameroon and took the virus, by ship, to German East Africa, on the other side of the continent (Figure 4.1).

When World War I broke out in 1914, the conflict was initially confined to Europe. Soon, however, the fighting spread to Africa, where French and British joint forces invaded German colonies. The first one to be lost by the Germans was Togo, in the first year of the war. Cameroon was lost in 1916, after two years of struggle. Meanwhile, South African troops conquered German Southwest Africa in 1915. After four years of fighting—the longest struggle for a colony—combined British and South African forces took German East Africa in 1918. These wars in Africa had a great impact on the local people. Villages were burned, which forced dislocation. Food supplies and labor forces were moved around by colonial powers, causing further dislocation and mixing of peoples. Most important, the Europeans used Africans in their colonial armies. The majority of soldiers on both sides of the African conflict were Africans. The colonial powers also recruited Africans to fight their battles in Europe.

At the end of World War I, German colonies were distributed among the victors. In 1919 the Belgians claimed Rwanda and Burundi; the British took the rest of East Africa. The French took 80 percent of Cameroon and Britain took 20 percent. By this time, HIV-1 was already seeded around Lake Victoria, where it would grow slowly into HIV-1A and the other African HIV-1 subtypes. But what about HIV-1B? The first cases of opportunistic PCP and cytomegalovirus (CMV) infections and tumors did not occur in Germany until 1939. If German colonists coming home after World War I brought proto-1B, we would expect such cases to occur in the 1920s. How do we account for the lag time?

Apparently those returning expatriates were not infected, or else they carried harmless strains of HIV. The potentially lethal proto-1B must have been imported later among about three hundred Germans who came home in 1939. These settlers had remained in Cameroon even though their land was confiscated. Within five years, they had repurchased their plantations from the British, at a London auction in 1924. The British had completely neglected Cameroon. Perhaps it did not seem worth the trouble, since their 20 percent was broken into the noncontiguous Southern and Northern Cameroons, lying respectively at the borders of Nigeria and French Cameroon. In any case, these German settlers regained all their possessions, only to lose them again after September 3, 1939, when war was declared between England and Germany. They repatriated rapidly that year, mostly by ship. Soon after their return, Germany saw its first fatal cases of PCP in the port city of Danzig, now Gdansk (Figure 4.2).

The Rise of African AIDS

Presumably, the HIV strain that came to Germany in 1939 was already able to cause disease, at least in low frequency, before it left Cameroon. What about the strains that left Cameroon at the turn of the century and migrated across central Africa?

This question is best answered by seeing if, and how frequently, AIDS-like cases occurred before recent times. If we look back, perhaps we can see when and how the current African epidemic took off. But pinpointing AIDS-like disease is not easy, especially in Africa. This is true today and was even more true in the past. After all, AIDS is not one disease but a collection of clinical manifestations that occur only because HIV has damaged the immune system. All known HIVs can cause this damage, but they rarely cause the diseases that follow. HIV has been established as the cause of certain dementias, and evidence is increasing that it causes certain diarrheas. But most AIDS-related diarrhea is caused by other agents, as are AIDS-related pneumonia and tumors. These other agents, such as *P. carinii* or herpesviruses, commonly infect people early in life but cause no harm if the immune system is healthy.

To spot AIDS we must look for unexpected or odd cases of pneumonia, diarrhea, or tumors. This is an easy task in Europe, where such problems were extremely rare before HIV emerged in the 1970s and 1980s. It is not easy in Africa, where such problems have long been common. Many

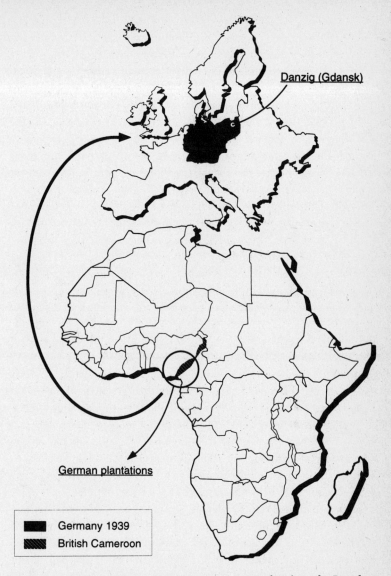

Danzig (Gdansk)

German plantations

Germany 1939
British Cameroon

Figure 4.2 **Travel of HIV-1 to Germany.** *German settlers from the British South Cameroons (a former German territory) could have brought the precursor of HIV-1B to Danzig. The first European AIDS cases occurred there in 1939, at the advent of World War II, when a number of settlers repatriated. This map of the time shows how they may have traveled by ship from Africa to the Baltic port.* (McEvedy 1980.)

Africans without HIV have Kaposi's sarcoma (KS), diarrhea, or wasting (i.e., severe weight loss) because their immune systems are compromised by malnutrition or multiple infections that have nothing to do with AIDS. Still, some sense can be made of the records, especially if we look at KS.

Kaposi's sarcoma is the most common tumor seen in Euro-American AIDS patients. It is a major risk not so much for HIV-positive hemophiliacs but for HIV-positive gay men. Of men infected by homosexual, or anal, transmission of HIV, one out of two gets KS, at least in Europe. The higher incidence among gay men suggests that orofecal contact, involved in some sexual practices, enhances the chance to acquire KS. Apparently feces can carry the agent that causes KS under circumstances including immune suppression and perhaps drug use. This agent has quite recently been identified as a herpesvirus. It can be detected in the KS lesions of virtually all patients, whether or not they are HIV-positive. The virus belongs to a group of herpes viruses known to multiply in white blood cells. It is not the group that includes the agents of genital herpes, herpes blisters, chicken pox, or shingles. Instead, the group includes Epstein-Barr virus, the agent of infectious mononucleosis, which also plays a causative role in certain blood cancers.

Beyond AIDS patients, KS is quite rare in the United States and Europe. It appears almost exclusively in two very distinct populations. By far the largest of these consists of gay men who are HIV-negative. They are affected much less often and less aggressively than gay men who are HIV-positive but far more than the general population. The appearance of KS in HIV-negative gay men again points to the risk of orofecal contact through homosexual relations. But KS also occurs, if rarely, in a population with no HIV or history of homosexuality: elderly men of Mediterranean, Middle Eastern, or Eastern European descent. So far, nobody can explain how these men acquired the KS agent or why they are susceptible.

Though rare in the Western world, KS has long been endemic in Africa. Its ubiquity makes it a tricky indicator of HIV or AIDS, but changes in KS frequency or severity may give us clues. Interestingly, Cameroon is the first African country from which it was reported. In 1914 a German doctor named Hallenberg described KS-like lesions in a Cameroonian man. Since then, many cases of severe and mild KS have been reported from many countries, particularly eastern and western Zaire, Rwanda and Burundi, western Uganda, and Tanzania. Kaposi's sarcoma was clearly endemic in these areas before AIDS appeared in the 1970s. Was an ancestral HIV allowing the KS agent to bloom, or did HIV have nothing to do with these early KS cases?

There is no way to be sure, since it was 1983 or 1984 before HIV was identified and we had good tests to assess immune function. Studies of the early 1970s suggest that, at that time, the most severe KS was sometimes, but not always, associated with immunological abnormalities. The earliest report is from Uganda in 1970. A 1973 report, using more refined technology, suggested that the most aggressive forms of KS were always linked with immunological abnormalities. However, as noted, in Africa such abnormalities can stem from many causes besides AIDS.

Once good testing was available, a study was conducted at the seven-hundred-bed Fomulac Hospital in Katana, Zaire, in 1984. The hospital's outpatient population included hundreds of thousands of residents on the eastern side of Lake Kivu, of whom 10 to 15 percent were already infected with HIV. The study found HIV in none of fourteen inpatients with KS but in two of twelve controls, that is, people without KS who were admitted for trauma or elective surgery. One must assume that if most Zairian cases of KS were not associated with HIV in 1984, earlier cases were probably not associated either.

Even more revealing studies were done in Uganda during the 1980s. They found that while the KS agent was clearly present before the 1970s, it had not yet joined with HIV to create an epidemic of aggressive KS. Ugandans diagnosed with KS between 1971 and 1975 showed no HIV antibodies when their frozen samples were later analyzed. The same was true for healthy controls bled during the study period. Taken together, these findings strongly indicate that, in Uganda and Zaire in the 1970s, HIV had not yet enhanced the aggressivity and transmissibility of the KS agent. They suggest that, as late as 1975, HIV had not yet entered Uganda at all.

A letter published in the *Lancet* in 1986 (Nahmias, 1986) gave evidence for human infection by HIV-1 in Kinshasa, Zaire, as early as 1959. Unfortunately, it reported finding the virus in only 1 of 672 samples taken in 1959. This serological result was not verified by testing the viral RNA, so one must wonder if that one positive sample was contaminated with HIV-1 during the 1986 analysis period. If so, we have no evidence that HIV-1, as we know it, existed in Zaire in 1959. Nor we can detect any sign of an AIDS-related epidemic at that time in Zaire.

However, we have good evidence that the picture had changed by the mid-1970s. HIV appears to have begun invasion of Zaire about that time. A form of HIV had evolved into a true AIDS virus by growing out to a true and recognizable subtype, similar to what is seen today in the same part of Africa. The first evidence is a letter published in the *Lancet* (Bygbjerg, 1983) describing a Danish surgeon who died in 1977, at age forty-seven, with signs suggestive of AIDS. This previously healthy woman had worked from 1972 to 1975 in a very primitive rural hospital in the north of Zaire. In 1976, after returning to her home country of Denmark, she developed intermittent diarrhea, fatigue, and wasting that were resistant to therapy. The next year she vacationed in South Africa, where she developed a severe acute pneumonia. Returning home in July 1977, she was diagnosed with PCP, oral candidiasis, and evidence of an acquired immunodeficiency. She died in December. Her case was the first evidence that a new kind of AIDS was emerging in Africa, one with such manifestations as PCP but also with new manifestations: severe diarrhea and wasting.

The year the surgeon died, similar cases of wasting disease began to appear in Kinshasa, the capital of Zaire. We do not know if HIV was present because in 1983, when these cases were reported, HIV testing was not yet widely available. But in 1985 the wasting disease was linked to HIV by a cluster of Rwandan cases. As reported in the *Lancet* (Jonckheer, 1985), they involved a Rwandan family of three young boys and their parents. Infected in the mid-1970s, all five of these people had some degree of immunodeficiency and tested HIV-positive. Particularly the twenty-nine-year-old mother suffered chronic diarrhea and severe weight loss. Apparently an HIV epidemic was emerging in rural Zaire and Rwanda, but its cause was an HIV variant not seen in the United States and Europe. This virus was associated primarily with diarrhea and wasting and only secondarily with symptoms like KS.

The virus was officially identified in 1987 through analysis of sera from a 1976 campaign to determine the prevalence of Ebola virus in Zaire. Of 454 serum samples preserved from that time, five were found positive for HIV. One was taken from a twenty-six-year-old woman living in a small town in northwestern Zaire. She had moved in 1971 to Kinshasa, returned to her hometown in 1975, and died in 1978 from severe diarrhea and weight loss. These problems were accompanied by what appeared to be pneumonia and oral candidiasis. In 1987 a virus was isolated from her 1976 serum sample and shown to be a strain of HIV-1. Subsequent sequence analysis further showed it was HIV-1 subtype A.

This 1976 isolate (strain HZ321) is our earliest actual sample of HIV, since no virus has yet been recovered from the Norway sailor. The isolate reveals three important things. First, HIV-1A had reached rural Zaire by 1976. Second, it had gained the ability to cause disease but one different from Western AIDS. Third, its aggressive nature proved the firm establishment of HIV-1 subtypes, or at least subtype A. If the common ancestor was harmless at the turn of the century, this evolutionary process had taken about seventy-five years.

The question remains, Did HIV-1 increase virulence by forming subtypes, or did it become virulent and then form subtypes during epidemic spread? For the answer we must ask another question: Did the Zairian HIV-1A isolate (HZ321) come from the west or the east? Presumably its twenty-six-year-old host was infected after 1975, whereas the Danish surgeon was infected between 1972 and 1975. The Rwandan cluster shows the virus was circulating in Rwanda in 1977. So by the mid-1970s, HIV-1 subtypes were apparently established, spreading west through central Africa and causing predominantly a wasting disease with high mortality. Unlike HIV-1B, the African HIV does not seem to have gone through an intermediate state of aggressivity. However, such a stage may have occurred but gone unnoticed in Africa because of the generally poor health and record keeping there.

Taken together, these points suggest that HIV-1 had to form subtypes to achieve the kind of disease frequency we see with AIDS. Each subtype consists of many strains that share certain defining characteristics, including optimal spread and an asymptomatic period. For example, all strains of HIV-1 subtype B spread optimally by anal intercourse and cause disease after a symptom-free period of about ten years.

What Spurred Subtype Development in Africa?

If the ancestral HIV-1 from Cameroon lay nearly dormant for decades, some change in the environment or population must have caused it to blossom into aggressive diarrhea-causing subtypes. This change most likely occurred where Uganda and Tanzania meet, west of Lake Victoria. In that area a new disease emerged in the early 1980s. Locally called "slim disease" because of its wasting effects, it was characterized by the diarrhea, weight loss, and fever seen in the Danish and Zairian women and the Rwandan family. On a 1985 field trip, a Ugandan team counted twenty-nine cases of "slim disease" in the Masaka and Rakai districts of rural Uganda, and every patient was HIV-positive. But the first recognized case of this disease occurred in a small town just inside Tanzania, at the shore of Lake Victoria. The disease seems to have come to Uganda from Tanzania, imported by traders and soldiers. In 1985, ten of fifteen Tanzanians who routinely traded across the Tanzanian-Ugandan border were shown to be HIV-positive. These traders had regular sexual interactions with the Ugandan villagers. They traded goods for sex with both men and women, but predominantly women, in a pattern that went back to the early 1970s.

That same period saw frequent military clashes on the Tanzanian-Ugandan border. In 1973 an agreement to end the hostilities was signed between Nyerere of Tanzania and General Idi Amin of Uganda. However, hostilities resumed in 1978 when Ugandan troops invaded northern Tanzania and the Tanzanian army counterattacked. In 1979 Tanzanian forces marched into Kampala, ousted Idi Amin, and remained in Uganda well into the 1980s. Many acts of violence—probably including sexual violence—were reportedly committed against the Ugandan people, especially in border areas. In addition to raping or consorting with Ugandan women, the soldiers no doubt attracted prostitutes, who have always been helpful in spreading sexually transmissible diseases such as AIDS.

So for half a century, African HIV-1 was transmitted only fast enough to sustain a low level of endemicity—not fast enough to increase its virulence. Then, in the late 1960s and early 1970s, it encountered new opportunities in rural areas of Uganda and northwestern Tanzania. Transmitted more rapidly by the mainly heterosexual activity of traders and particularly soldiers, the virus formed the well-documented HIV-1A and other subtypes adept at heterosexual transmission. Morbidity and mortality increased in the process. The subtypes then spread their lethal wasting syndrome beyond Uganda and Tanzania, launching the outbreak of AIDS in Africa in last half of the 1970s.

One might ask why so many HIV-1 subtypes formed in a relatively small area, all causing the same disease. The answer is that the virus was apparently nonpathogenic or very weak when imported from Cameroon to German East Africa. Unlike the "proto-1B" that went to Europe in 1939, the

African precursor had no evolutionary direction when it met its opportunity for increased transmission. Its nature was (and remains) to infect a host, then rapidly to form a swarm of genetically linked, yet distinct, virus clones. Following sexual transmission, one of these clones is selected by its ability to survive in the new host. However, in some cases, the selected variant can infect the host but causes little or no disease. As explained in Chapter 1, the crucial factor is virus load: the better a virus replicates in a host, the more rapidly the virus is transmitted and the more rapidly the next host develops disease. Initially, before the African HIV-1 grew into subtypes, there was as much or more variation among strains as now exists among subtypes. Out of an enormous swarm of HIV-1 variants, all those ill adapted to heterosexual spread gradually disappeared. This left only the most well-adapted progeny, including the A, C, and D subtypes (Figure 4.3a,b,c).

Another reason for the formation of multiple HIV-1 subtypes may be the health condition of African hosts. As we know, HIV-1 replicates best

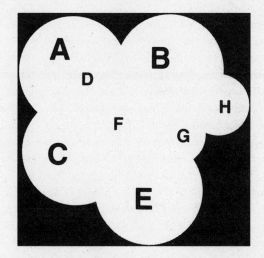

Figure 4.3a   **Formation of HIV-1 subtypes in RNA sequence space**. *In RNA sequence space, the viral universe conceived by Nobelist Manfred Eigen, related but nonidentical virus populations follow their trajectory as "swarms" with one master sequence as the center of gravity. In the beginning, the subtypes were barely distinguishable members of the HIV-1 family.* (Lukashov and Goudsmit 1996)

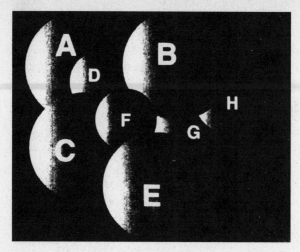

Figure 4.3b   *As the Western and African AIDS epidemics arose, the subtypes gained definition.* (Lukashov and Goudsmit 1996)

when its host cells are activated. Activation occurs when the immune system is alerted by invasion of foreign organisms or substances, or the resulting infection. Invasion by parasites (as in malaria), bacteria (as in typhus), and viruses (as in hepatitis) is only too common in Africa. All of these invaders activate white blood cells or T cells, including the CD4+ cells that attract HIV. The more these cells are activated when HIV appears, the more likely HIV is to establish a widespread infection with multiple strains.

When women newly infected with HIV-1 were studied in Rwanda, they were found to differ in two important ways from people newly infected in the United States and Europe. Euro-American infections show the multiplication of a genetically homogeneous virus population of HIV-1B. In contrast, infections in Rwanda start out with heterogeneous virus populations of HIV-1A, and some new infections start with recombinant viruses whose parents are HIV-1A and C. One woman studied was infected with both a parental A strain and an A/C recombinant strain.

As we know, recombinants do not occur easily. To produce an A/C recombinant, one cell needs to be infected by both A and C viruses. The particular strains must share enough genes to permit crossover of genetic in-

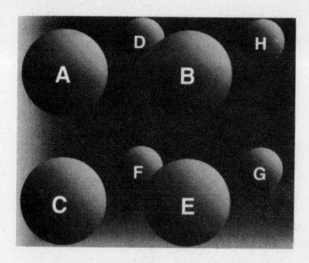

Figure 4.3c *As the epidemics progress, the subtypes show increasing definition and interstrain variation but do not merge.* (Lukashov and Goudsmit 1996)

formation. Then, from their mating, heterozygotes are produced with the genetic information of A on one RNA strand and C on the other. These infect new cells and mate, producing homozygous offspring in which A and C genetic information has crossed over from one RNA strand to another. These offspring are recombinants, each having two identical RNA strands composed of mixed A/C genes (Figure 3.2).

The higher state of T cell activation in African hosts may well be the main reason why multiple HIV-1 subtypes are so rapidly formed in Africa. Yet after their formation, they remain recognizable subtypes despite strain variation that increases in the course of an epidemic. As integrity is preserved in HIV-1B after ten to fifteen years of the Amsterdam epidemic, so it is preserved in HIV-1A after almost twenty years of spread in Africa. This phenomenon can only be explained by virulence equilibrium. HIV-1 subtypes are directly linked to the course of infection in humans, that is, an asymptomatic period just long enough to transmit the virus to others by some sexual route.

From the time HIV-1 was seeded in the former German East Africa, about 1900, to the emergence of "slim disease" in what are now Uganda and Tanzania, the virus probably created far more variants than it has since 1975. Many of those early variants died out from lack of transmission. Some failed because of too little infectivity. Others failed because of too much: they grew so fast to such high titers, or levels, that the host sickened and died before he or she could transmit the virus to a new host. The current HIV-1 subtypes were created by decades of constant elimination of too-weak or too-strong variants from the pool.

This process continues, so we can predict that subtypes may disappear from a given locale if they are too aggressive to allow the host time for sexual activity. Indeed, we have preliminary evidence that this is happening right now in Uganda, an area dominated by HIV-1 subtypes A and D, whose shares of infections were initially about equal. But it seems that subtype D is more aggressive than the other known subtypes. It replicates to enormously high levels at the moment of acute infection and maintains this high virus load, causing AIDS to occur in a few years instead of a decade. We now see this subtype becoming less and less prevalent. Its history seems to support the idea that a virus can be too aggressive—too successful at killing its host—to survive in a population.

Distribution by Truck Routes

Once HIV-1 subtypes were established just west of Lake Victoria, these agents and their wasting variant of AIDS began to fan out (Figure 4.4). Mainly subtypes A and C spread along the north-south axis and the east-west axis. HIV-1A favored the latter, becoming the predominant subtype from Kenya in the east to Cameroon and Ivory Coast in the west. HIV-1C has traveled the other axis, flourishing from Ethiopia in the Horn of Africa to Zambia, Malawi, and South Africa. The two axes of HIV-1 distribution tend to follow the rain forest. More to the point, they follow the roads through the rain forest, which head out from Lake Victoria in all directions. These are used mainly by trucks since cars are scarce.

Of course, HIV is not carried by roads or trucks. It is carried by people: the truckers who drive the routes in relay, and the prostitutes or village women they meet along the way. Starting at Mombasa and Dar es Salaam

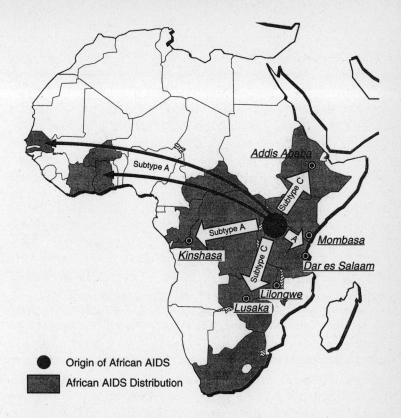

Figure 4.4 Spread of main African subtypes. *HIV-1 subtype A has followed routes running east from Lake Victoria to Mombasa and Dar es Salaam and west as far as Kinshasa in Zaire. It most likely reached West Africa by air travel between francophone countries (see black-tipped arrows). HIV-1C has followed truck routes north to Addis Ababa and south to Lilongwe and Lusaka (see white arrows).*

on the eastern coast, two main east-west routes link Nairobi in Kenya, Kampala in Uganda, Kigali in Rwanda, Kinshasa in Zaire, and cities farther west. North-south routes run to Addis Ababa in Ethiopia and down to Lilongwe in Malawi and Lusaka in Zambia.

   If the virus has traveled these routes, we should find two kinds of evidence. First, the truckers who live and work nearest to Lake Victoria should be infected at the highest rate, compared with truckers who live and work in outlying areas. Second, the prevalence of infection along the routes should be highest in individuals and villages closest to the truck routes, compared with those farther from the routes. Both types of evidence have been documented. More than half of Rwandan truck drivers are HIV-1 positive, compared with about a third of Ugandan drivers and about a fifth of those in Kenya or Ethiopia. Similarly, in the early 1990s, most prostitutes of the interior were infected, compared with half of those in Ethiopia. And the farther a village population lived from a truck route, the lower its percentage of HIV-1 infections.

So we now have the final piece of the puzzle. According to the scenario proposed in this chapter, HIV-1 arose in Cameroon and was carried to German East Africa about 1900, and to Germany in 1939. HIV-1B adapted to spread by anal intercourse, causing the Western AIDS epidemic. In Africa, HIV-1 viruses adapted to spread by vaginal intercourse, launching AIDS epidemics on that continent. They caused the African wasting form of AIDS by forming subtypes, mainly 1A and 1C. Sometimes called "slim disease," African AIDS arose in northern Tanzania west of Lake Victoria in the early 1970s. It spread to neighboring Uganda, Rwanda, and Zaire in the late 1970s. From there, along rain forest truck routes, HIV-1A spread east and west, while HIV-1C spread north and south.

But more puzzles remain. If the ancestral HIV-1 arose in Cameroon, how and where did this event occur? If the virus was initially harmless, how and why did it gain virulence as it went from human to human?

5

HIV-0 and HIV-1: The Chimpanzee Connection

We have proposed that the former German colony of Cameroon is the birthplace of HIV-1, the main cause of AIDS around the world. This idea gains strength from the fact that the same area is quite clearly the birthplace of HIV-0. Closely related to HIV-1, this virus is less well known because it has stayed close to home, infecting only a few people in Cameroon and Gabon. Its discovery was published in 1990 by van der Groen and Piot of the Institute of Tropical Medicine (ITM) in Antwerp.

A year earlier, a nineteen-year-old teacher from Cameroon felt ill while visiting Belgium for a brushup course. Testing at the ITM found she had antibodies to HIV-1. The ITM also tested a sample from March 1987, on file for this teacher, which showed she was positive at that time. The next finding was a big surprise. When isolated, her virus strain (Ant 70) was clearly not HIV-2 but also did not look like HIV-1. If it was an HIV-1 strain, it was the most divergent ever seen. Still, the immune response of the Cameroonian teacher suggested this virus was related to HIV-1. In the confusion, the discovery was first called HIV-3. Techniques of genetic analysis were unsophisticated and slow compared with those used now, but when analysis was complete, the virus was renamed HIV-1 subgroup O. The O stood for "outgroup" because it seemed like a subgroup but also an outsider. The virus is better called HIV-0, with 0 meaning "zero." This name more appropriately describes the relationship to HIV-1, as is revealed in Chapter 3 and will be further illustrated in this chapter.

After Ant 70 had been isolated from the teacher, her Cameroonian husband was called in and found to harbor a very similar strain, Ant 70-NA. When the Belgians published these discoveries in 1990, the scientific community was perplexed. What kind of virus was this? Could it be the ancestor of all HIV-1 viruses? How did these two individuals get this strange infection? Would it progress to AIDS and cause death?

The last question was answered from Munich, Germany, where researchers isolated a third HIV-0 strain in collaboration with the University of Yaoundé in Cameroon. The Germans had obtained the strain in 1991 from a woman who had always lived in Cameroon. Her AIDS-related death in 1992 proved the new virus was a full-fledged member of the lethal HIV family.

The German group reported that HIV-0 circulated only in Cameroon and Gabon. It was not spotted in nearby Ivory Coast or Malawi, nor in Germany. The Belgian group subsequently showed that HIV-0 was not the cause of AIDS in Brazil, Belgium, or the African countries of Niger, Zaire, Kenya, or Rwanda. It soon became clear that even where HIV-0 causes AIDS, as in its home area, it is far from the leading cause. Of all HIV-positive individuals in Cameroon and Gabon, only a handful are infected with this virus. Moreover, HIV-0 apparently caused no AIDS in Cameroon before HIV-1 started the AIDS epidemic in central Africa. At least in urban areas (where the only testing has been conducted), HIV-0 seems to have emerged at about the same time as HIV-1. From the beginning, it caused infection and AIDS in far fewer people than HIV-1. In fact, documented cases are so scarce that, even in the mid-1990s, we can say little about this virus. It apparently remained confined to Cameroon and Gabon throughout the 1980s, even when HIV-1 subtypes began to spread rapidly along the African truck routes. Only in the 1990s did HIV-0 creep into West Africa and Europe; even then, all cases could be linked to Cameroon or Gabon. The most recent observations from France, the country with most European cases, confirm that HIV-0 can cause AIDS. But outside of France, HIV-0 has caused scarcely any infections in Europe. They have been seen only in people from Cameroon or Gabon or in people intimate with them. A single HIV-0 case has so far been reported in a Cameroonian immigrant in the United States.

So HIV-0, HIV-1, and HIV-2 all are AIDS viruses. Based on genetic comparisons, HIV-0 and HIV-1 are close relatives, and each is much closer to the other than to HIV-2. One might say that HIV-1 and HIV-0 are brother and sister, while HIV-2 is some sort of a nephew. The first two often overlap in the same geographic areas, but HIV-2 has not overlapped with them until recently (Figures 5.1 and 5.2). It has stayed in West Africa, where it probably arose in Benin: in the rain forest west of the Dahomey Gap. HIV-1 originated east of the Dahomey Gap (a stretch of savanna or grassland that divides the rain forest), most likely in the rain forests of Cameroon—exactly the home base of HIV-0. Can their shared locale be an amazing coincidence, or does it point to a shared ancestor? Could one be the ancestor of the other?

HIV-1 apparently needed export from Cameroon to East Africa, Europe, and the United States to evolve into an AIDS-causing virus. HIV-0 evolved to cause AIDS without leaving home. Since HIV-1 was reintroduced to Cameroon, it has become the leading cause of AIDS there, as in other African countries. Subtype A predominates, with a minor contribution by subtypes E, F, and H. HIV-1B has so far been identified in only one symptom-free individual. As already noted, HIV-0 viruses seem to have entered urban parts of Cameroon at the same time as HIV-1, or slightly later. The two have now merged in the Cameroon epidemic.

But if HIV-1 needed export to heat up and HIV-0 did not, these two closely related viruses must have encountered different circumstances during their rain forest stage of development. If multiple transmissions, from one human to another, are needed to create a true AIDS virus, HIV-0 must have begun to circulate earlier than HIV-1.

Let us go back to the nonhuman source, or reservoir, of these two related viruses. Can we trace this original host? There must have been a host, as viruses are parasites. They can infect or colonize any living thing, but viruses that infect bacteria or plants cannot also infect animal cells. So HIV came from an animal host. Indeed, HIV-like viruses are known to infect cows, house cats, lions, horses, sheep, goats, and various monkeys. Of these, close relatives of HIV are bovine immunodeficiency virus (BIV), feline immunodeficiency virus (FIV), equine infectious anemia virus (EIAV), and simian immunodeficiency virus (SIV). All named by analogy with HIV,

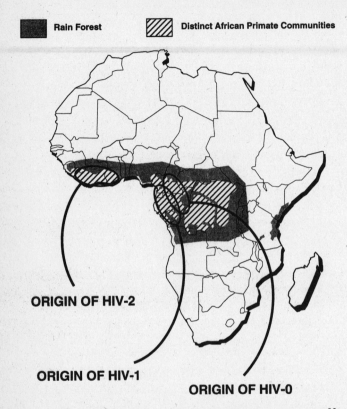

Figure 5.1   **Rise of HIV types in the central African rain forest**. *Hatching defines communities of nonhuman primates in (left to right) Upper Guinea, Cameroon, the western equatorial rain forest, Congo basin, and eastern Zaire, areas that support 80 percent of all forest monkeys and apes in Africa. HIV-2 arose in the Upper Guinea rain forest. Both HIV-0 and HIV-1 arose in the west-ern equatorial rain forest.* (Lee, Thornback, and Bennett 1988; Sayer, Harcourt, and Collins 1992.)

they cause little or no immunodeficiency in their natural hosts. Only EIAV and FIV cause clinical disease. (See Figure 8.1, lentivirus family tree.)

SIVs are closest of all to HIV, which is not surprising since monkeys, apes, and humans belong to the same primate family. The SIV of sooty

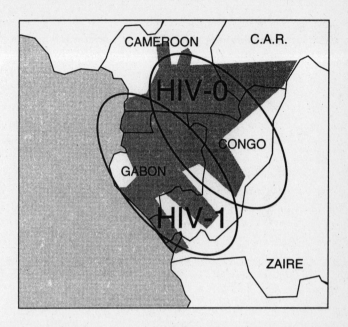

Figure 5.2   **Nonhuman primate community of the western equatorial rain forest**. *Although their regions overlap, HIV-1 appears to have arisen in the Gabonese part of the rain forest, whereas HIV-0 arose in the less accessible inland region bordered by western Zaire, southern Central African Republic, eastern Cameroon, northern Congo, and northeastern Gabon.* (Janssens et al. 1994; deLeys et al. 1990; Peeters et al. 1992.)

mangabeys (SIV sm) is extremely close to HIV-2 but less close to HIV-0 and HIV-1. Remarkably, HIV-2 is more like this virus of West African monkeys than like HIV-0 and HIV-1. As discussed in Chapter 6, this implies that HIV-2—but not the other AIDS viruses—is directly and recently descended from its SIV ancestor. The West African sooty mangabeys may well be the past and present source animal for the West African HIV-2.

Could some other monkey or ape be the source animal for HIV-0 and HIV-1? Ever since AIDS emerged, researchers have favored this possibility but, despite much speculation, had no promising leads until the late 1980s. Then van der Groen and Piot decided to take action. Suspecting chimpanzees, they tested fifty wild-caught animals for HIV, hoping to detect SIV. Captured in different parts of the rain forest of Gabon, the chimpanzees were largely adult animals housed in the Primate Center of Gabon in Franceville. Only two animals, both preadult females, tested seropositive. They were infected but showed no sign of disease. The first, born in the rain forest of northwestern Gabon, was captured at six months by hunters who had shot her mother. (Unfortunately, commercial hunters usually kill the mother, as chimpanzees are extremely dangerous when defending their young.) The animal was acquired as a pet by a European family who lived in Gabon. The second seropositive chimpanzee was captured at age two when hunters killed her mother in the rain forest of northeast Gabon. The young animal was wounded and died a week later, so her virus was not isolated.

However, the virus of the first young chimpanzee was isolated in Antwerp. To encourage virus multiplication and facilitate isolation, infected cells from the animal were grown for ten days with uninfected human or chimpanzee white blood cells. Once isolated, the virus was labeled SIV cpz-gab1 (i.e., first chimpanzee strain from Gabon) and examined by electron microscopy. Enlarged thirty-five thousand times, the virus looked like a member of the HIV/SIV family, but more exact proof was needed.

As we know, individuals infected with HIV generate antibodies that react (i.e., recognize and bind) to certain proteins of those viruses. Some antibodies react to envelope proteins embedded in the viral coat. Others react to proteins at the inner core of the virus particle. HIV/SIV viruses vary widely in their envelope proteins but share many core proteins, conserved from the common ancestor.

When antibodies to core proteins of one virus react to those of other viruses, this cross-reaction proves family relationship. Studies have shown, for example, that HIV antibodies react to core proteins from the SIVs of sooty mangabeys and mandrills (SIV sm and SIV mnd). Studies in our lab have shown that sera of HIV-infected individuals react to the core protein of EIAV, a lentivirus of horses, but not to the proteins of lentiviruses of sheep and goats. This closeness of HIV and SIV to EIAV has provided an important clue to the family history that will be discussed in Chapter 8.

So the Belgian group expected that HIV-1 and HIV-2 antibodies would react to core proteins of SIV cpz-gab1, and they were right. However, whereas antibodies to both HIVs recognized its core proteins, only HIV-1 antibodies recognized the envelope proteins of SIV cpz-gab 1. Their signatures were nearly identical, showing very close relationship and even suggesting that SIV cpz was the ancestor of HIV-1.

The Belgians subsequently found that core proteins of SIV cpz-gab1 were recognized by antibodies in sera of a mandrill infected with SIV mnd. However, the core proteins were not recognized by antibodies in sera of an African green monkey infected with SIV agm. To complete the story, these researchers then reversed the experiment. They asked themselves if sera from the infected chimpanzee would react with proteins of HIV-1 and HIV-2 and SIV mnd and SIV agm. They found that chimpanzee sera bound firmly to both core and envelope proteins of HIV-1. It bound only to core proteins of HIV-2, SIV mnd, and SIV agm. This provides strong evidence that SIV cpz is closer to HIV-1 than to HIV-2, and that SIV cpz and HIV-1 have the same origin—or that one originated from the other.

The Belgians made several striking discoveries. First, SIV cpz-gab1 was closest to HIV-1 of all HIVs and SIVs then known. Second, this Gabonese SIV was only distantly related to HIV-2 and SIV mnd. Third, the SIV of sooty mangabeys was closer to SIV agm than to SIV cpz or SIV mnd. Final proof of the pudding came from preliminary genetic analysis. If seen as a strain of HIV-1, SIV cpz-gab1 was highly divergent in the same way as HIV-0 but still within the family, just as SIV sm and HIV-2 are within the same family.

The identification of SIV cpz-gab1 immediately launched a heated debate. Two hypotheses were advanced to explain the closeness of SIV cpz and HIV-1. A skeptical camp argued that this SIV was really a human virus. Either the Belgian group had inadvertently contaminated its cultures with HIV or the chimpanzee baby was infected on capture by an HIV-positive hunter. This skepticism was based on the fact that so few seropositive chimpanzees had been found (only two of fifty), and only one strain had been isolated.

However, the other camp argued the exciting hypothesis that SIV cpz-gab1 was actually the ancestor of HIV-1. It had a very plausible explanation for why only two of fifty chimpanzees were SIV-positive. In general, adult chimpanzees cannot be captured alive without great danger, so hunters usually capture very young animals. Since we know that vervets, grivets, and other monkeys are SIV-infected only after reproductive age, this may well be the case with chimpanzees. Although the fifty chimpanzees were

between two and fifteen years old, virtually all were captured before reproductive age so, naturally, few were SIV-infected.

This argument may sound convincing, but the scientific community
wanted more testing of viruses and chimpanzees, so the Belgians complied.
Their next sample included forty-four wild-caught chimpanzees living in
Belgium or the zoo of Abidjan, Ivory Coast. Luckily, one chimpanzee tested
seropositive for HIV antibodies, showing SIV infection. He was a young
male, approximately four years old, who had been brought illegally to
Belgium from Zaire as a pet. When seized by customs officials at the Brussels airport, he was two or three years old. When his virus was isolated in
Antwerp, it was called SIV cpz-ant. It was closely related to SIV cpz-gab1—
but how closely? If too close, skeptics would dismiss both viruses as Belgian contaminations in the laboratory. Was the second virus different
enough to confirm circulation of SIV cpz strains in the wild?

Evidence against lab contamination included the fact that the young
male with SIVcpz-ant landed at Brussels with a two-year-old male that was
seronegative. Ever since their confiscation, these two males have been in-
separable cage-mates, but the seronegative animal has remained so. If lab
contamination had occurred, it probably would have affected both animals.
The two chimpanzees have now shared a cage for seven years, but the virus
has not been transmitted in saliva, urine, feces, or even in blood exchanged
during their occasional scuffles. Apparently only sex transmits this virus in
nature, and the male with SIV cpz-ant was never introduced to the female
with SIV cpz-gab1. So it seemed the seropositive male had been infected in
the wild, but suspicion remained, especially since both SIVcpz viruses had
been isolated in the same laboratory. Finally, comparison of the viral genes
ended all speculation. It showed that all the Belgian SIV cpz and HIV-0
viruses were independent isolates, clearly related but distinct enough that
all must be genuine.

A few years later, the Belgian work was further confirmed by independent researchers working in the United States. They were headed by Beatrice Hahn, who had left Gallo's lab for the University of Alabama at Birm-
ingham. Her group found a third chimpanzee virus now called SIV cpz-us.
Its host had died, so the virus could not be isolated, but genetic analysis of
viral gene fragments from postmortem tissue showed that this chimpanzee
virus was closely related to the two others and to HIV-1 and HIV-0 strains.

About this same time, the Belgians performed genetic analysis on gene
fragments from the second Gabonese chimpanzee—the one that died of

wounds a week after her capture in Africa. They identified a strain called SIV cpz-gab2, bringing the grand total to four.

These findings should convince everybody that SIV circulates among chimpanzees in the wild, and that these viruses are harmless to the chimpanzee despite their close relationship to HIV-1 and HIV-0 viruses. Unfortunately, the chimpanzee studied by the Hahn group has a mysterious background. Nobody knows where it came from, and persistent skeptics have suggested that this chimpanzee, along with the Belgian chimpanzees, was not infected by SIV but by HIV acquired through inoculation with human blood.

This is actually not as far-fetched as it sounds. In the 1950s and 1960s, especially in Zaire, commercial hunters routinely inoculated newly captured baby chimpanzees with human blood to vaccinate these valuable animals against human diseases. The skeptics claim that such practices introduced HIV to chimpanzees, who now circulate the virus as SIV. This idea deserves mention but seems extremely unlikely, given the genetic distance between the HIV and the chimpanzee viruses. The SIV cpz-ant and SIV cpz-gab1 and 2 isolates show too much interstrain variation to have branched from HIV just a few decades ago.

Ironically, the fact that blood and blood-borne disease can be exchanged between chimpanzees and humans is most extensively documented by the very institution that gave us the first SIV cpz and HIV-0 isolates: the ITM in Antwerp. Between 1935 and 1955, ITM researchers inoculated humans with malaria-infected monkey and ape blood in order to study the transmissibility of malaria to humans. Like other scientists in the past, they sometimes conducted human experimentation by ethics that now seem primitive. Human subjects were sometimes prisoners or patients with mental retardation or terminal disease. For the ITM malaria studies, most subjects were individuals suffering from dementia praecox or paraplegia due to late-stage syphilis.

Initially, these people were inoculated with blood from malaria-infected Asian monkeys (rhesus macaques), but the animals did not transmit their disease. So the researchers switched to apes and, in 1939, injected people with large volumes of malaria-infected chimpanzee blood (up to 15 milliliters). Finally, in 1955, they reported the following chimpanzee-human-chimpanzee blood passage experiment.

A female chimpanzee two to three years old, captured in Wamba, North Zaire, was found to be infected with chimpanzee malaria when she arrived at the Antwerp zoo on October 18, 1954. Two weeks later, blood from this chimpanzee was injected into a second chimpanzee, infecting her with malaria. Then a twenty-five-year-old man and an eighteen-year-old woman were inoculated with 4.5 cc of blood from the second chimpanzee. Two months after inoculation, the man had two bouts of malarial fever, but the woman remained malaria-free. During the man's second attack, 7 cc of his blood was taken and injected into a fifty-seven-year-old man. This man got malaria much quicker. Less than one week after receiving the infected blood, he suffered fourteen bouts of malarial fever. Blood taken during one of his first attacks was injected into three additional men, all in their fifties, and also into one chimpanzee. The chimpanzee and two of the men got malaria. Blood of one of the infected men was injected into a woman of twenty-seven, who also got malaria. Blood from the chimpanzee was then injected into a man and woman, both in their forties. As might be expected, these subjects got malaria. Incredibly, the series of studies ended with in-oculation of infected blood from the man in his forties into an elderly man who was completely healthy. He had just retired from a career in the Bel-gian Congo (now Zaire).

Aside from their dubious ethics of human experimentation, these early Belgian studies risked causing an epidemic. If any SIV or HIV had been present in just one human or chimpanzee subject, it would surely have been transmitted from chimpanzee to human, or vice versa. In Amsterdam we documented that 10 to 100 microliters of HIV-infected blood is enough to transmit HIV with high efficiency. Those Belgian experiments involved injection of fifty to two hundred times as much blood. In the early 1980s, Nobelist D. Carleton Gajdusek injected more than fifty chimpanzees with HIV and blood from AIDS patients. Virtually all of the chimpanzees be-came infected, which confirms that both humans and chimpanzees are highly susceptible to blood-borne HIV infection, and little virus is needed to initiate an infection when virus is brought in contact with susceptible blood cells.

Reportedly, none of the people involved in the Belgian experiments be-came terminally ill, although follow-up was short. The same studies, if done in Zaire, could well have resulted in the spread of SIV or HIV in a new species. Also, the studies were frighteningly well suited to cycle a relatively innocent virus into a harmful virus. Fortunately, the time or place was not fertile for an epidemic. These studies cannot be blamed for helping to spread AIDS, but they show how naive researchers could be. Perhaps their best excuse is that no dramatic outbreaks had occurred at that time. No Ebola or AIDS had yet been reported. Researchers simply had no idea of these threats. In fact, given antibiotics and other recent discoveries, they had a false sense of security and power over nature. The Belgian malaria experiments have not been implicated in the rise of HIV or AIDS in Europe, but they remind us that infectious outbreaks can sometimes be more man-made than we would like to think. They remind us that science, like all human effort, can have a dark side despite all good intentions.

Let us return to the bright side: the Belgian discoveries of SIV cpz and HIV-0. If we need more evidence linking chimpanzee SIV to HIV-0 and HIV-1, we can look at the distribution overlap of the three SIV cpz viruses of known provenance. Two came from the northern rain forest of Gabon; the third came from Zaire. If their ancestors were transmitted to humans in the central African rain forest, we might assume a common time frame, location, and circumstances for these events that gave rise to HIV-1 and HIV-0. But while these two HIV types are closely related, they are also quite different. When we look at their genes, we see that all HIV-1 viruses cluster together and apart from all HIV-0 viruses. This strongly suggests that each type has been through a lot of changes since the two branched apart. They also differ biologically. HIV-1 viruses take two distinct forms: one geared for better transmissibility, and one geared for faster disease progression (the large syncytial cells mentioned earlier). HIV-0 has these two forms plus a third intermediate form.

We must conclude that transmission of HIV-1 and HIV-0 did not occur in the same time frame, locale, and circumstances. Although the family histories of these viruses are similar, they differ in crucial ways. One may speculate that HIV-0 was transmitted in a rain forest area with little exposure to the outside world but with enough inhabitants to permit slow and local evolution into an AIDS virus. HIV-1 was also transmitted in the rain forest, but later, in a fringe area. The event occurred at a time and place conducive to inroads by visitors who might become infected, then carry the virus to urban areas.

The fact that some chimpanzee strains cluster with HIV-1 and others with HIV-0 points to more than one transmission event. Chimpanzees may have passed the virus directly to humans, but this actually seems doubtful given the very low rate of HIV circulation among modern chimpanzees in the wild. Perhaps a third monkey, such as the colobus, was prey for both humans and chimpanzees and passed the virus to both of them at about the same time.

Two Distinct Rain Forest Ecosystems

To explain the distinctions between HIV-0 and HIV-1, one must postulate two distinct ecosystems that have no contact. The HIV-0 habitat must have contained an isolated tribe of forest people (also called pygmies, a name they dislike) and a troop of chimpanzees. This ecosystem was cut off from the outside world until recently, when forest people began to move to urban areas. Likewise, the HIV-1 habitat must have contained forest people and chimpanzees; however, it was close enough to the outside world that visitors sometimes intruded.

Such distinct ecosystems are readily found in this region of Africa, even when the rain forest is relatively continuous and not interrupted by patches of savanna. Forest people are distributed across nine African countries, including Cameroon and Gabon, but they often keep to themselves, in groups separated by geography and culture. In rain forest areas, these people are often completely unaware of neighboring groups just a short distance away. Yet in their separate territories, the forest people often live harmoniously, as hunter-gatherers, with African seminomads who farm the forest fringes. In fact, intermarriage is not infrequent.

Like the forest people, various nonhuman primates are scattered throughout the rain forest in distinct and noncontiguous territories. For example, gorillas are found in just two areas of rain forest, even though the areas between are perfectly suitable to their needs. A common explanation is that, in arid times, the animals stayed within the receding forest and, when times improved, were slow to follow when the forest flowed back.

Chimpanzees share territory with forest people but keep their distance. Two main factors determine chimpanzee distribution and survival: the absence of humans and the presence of food, fruit in particular. Chimpanzees need large quantities of fruit throughout the year. They are therefore threatened not only by poachers but by farmers who clear land by burning chimpanzee resources.

Chimpanzee troops number twenty to one hundred individuals and range over 10 to 200 square kilometers. They generally retreat from hu-

mans and, in the past, rarely saw or attacked humans. They were tradition-
ally hunted for food, but contact has now intensified because they are
hunted—with guns—mainly for export to zoos. One may safely assume
that contact began to increase in the late nineteenth century, when Europeans occupied most of Africa. Since Europeans explored the rain forest
and fancied animals as pets and zoological curiosities, they may well be the
visitors who brought HIV-1 back to urban areas.

However, HIV-0 began evolution much earlier than HIV-1. The virus
has not yet been found among forest people, but its introduction among
them seems not only plausible but inevitable. It would naturally follow
from the requirements of local human survival. Most forest people eat
monkey and ape meat and have probably done so for hundreds of years.
Like other apes, chimpanzees are large and active mostly during the day,
which makes them relatively easy hunting targets. Yet forest people have always risked injury from chimpanzees. Especially in the past, before they
had guns, they could easily be infected by SIV when bitten by an animal.
They could also be infected by eating raw or improperly cooked chimpanzee meat. (Within a species, both SIV and HIV are transmitted sexually, but from one species to another, e.g., ape to human, the virus must
spread in saliva or blood, since cross-species sex is rarely an option.)

The preceding scenarios could explain why HIV-0 and HIV-1 were introduced to humans in different parts of the rain forest and had quite different histories of circulation and spread (Figures 5.1 and 5.2). Can we
pinpoint more closely the probable location of the original transmission
events? Much circumstantial evidence is available.

Of the four documented SIV cpz viruses, the two Gabonese strains are
closer to HIV-1 than to HIV-0. This suggests that HIV-1 might have come
from a cross-species transmission in the rain forest of the Cameroon-
Gabon border region. As already noted, Cameroon under German rule was
the most likely source of the HIV-1 virus that started the AIDS epidemic
west of Lake Victoria in the 1970s. Meanwhile, the British Cameroons
were the most likely origin of the HIV-1 virus that went to Germany in
1939. The British Cameroons were separated into North Cameroons and
South Cameroons. If the two Gabonese strains came from the north of
Gabon, they were most likely transmitted (by chimpanzees or some other
monkey) in the western and coastal area of the western equatorial rain forest that borders modern Gabon, Cameroon, and the Congo. The ancestor
of HIV-1 must have been transported from that rain forest to the forest area

of South Cameroons, where most German settlers had their plantations between 1924 and 1939. This area is quite accessible to visitors.

The Alabama strain, SIV cpz-us, is closer to HIV-0 than to HIV-1 or the two Gabonese strains. Again, this suggests that cross-species transmission of HIV-1 and HIV-0 took place under different circumstances. We still do not know the provenance of the chimpanzee source of the Alabama SIV, but the very restricted circulation area of HIV-0 points to a Cameroonian origin. If the original transmission occurred in a relatively inaccessible area that supports both forest people and chimpanzees, we favor the eastern part of the west equatorial rainforest. This area includes the eastern tip of Cameroon, the northern Congo, and the western part of the Central African Republic.

Can we tell when these transmission events occurred? Once HIV-0 was passed to humans, it needed time to generate both extensive strain variation and the ability to cause AIDS. For a virus limited to sexual transmission within a small population, such as the forest people, this evolution would take many viral and host generations. Only after HIV-1 had reached epidemic proportions, in the early 1980s, did we notice HIV-0 and its ability to cause AIDS. Had it just gained this ability? Or had people from the remote eastern part of the west equatorial rain forest just begun to enter urban areas? The latter seems more likely. Otherwise we have the amazing coincidence that HIV-0 suddenly evolved to virulence just when HIV-1 began to spread along truck routes. Probably HIV-0 appeared in urban Cameroon simply because, in recent decades, rural people all over Africa have been moving toward the cities. It most likely became an AIDS virus in seclusion, a process requiring at least two to four hundred years, or eight to sixteen human generations, after the first transmission from chimpanzee or monkey.

A similar time frame might well apply to HIV-1 except that it reached urban areas faster, having come from a more accessible part of the rain forest. But a few HIV-1 strains evidently became virulent much sooner than others, notably the one that went to Germany in 1939. If such precocious strains caused terminal disease before the current epidemic took off—even at relatively low frequency—why was AIDS not reported long before it was? Probably the main reason is that until the end of the last century, these rain forest areas were virtually unexplored by outsiders. Local people undoubtedly explored them, but conveyed no information to the world at large. Only when outsiders arrived did a rain forest virus have the chance to emerge and be noticed, much less to cause an epidemic in a large number of people.

By the eighteenth century, African coastal areas and deserts were visited by outsiders to Africa. Since the Middle Ages, Arabs had used the desert roads and reported on their travels, especially trips to the Sudan. Europeans had settlements on the western coast as early as the fifteenth century. They initially traded exotic products, then slaves. They circumnavigated Africa in the sixteenth century and encountered the Arabs, who stayed mainly in eastern coastal areas. However, the early European and Arab merchants saw no reason to penetrate the east or west African interior. Later, even when the eastern and southern parts of the continent saw intrusion in the early nineteenth century, the west remained hidden.

In 1842 the French established an outpost at the mouth of the Ogooué River in Gabon. In the late 1850s the French-American Paul du Chaillu apparently entered the rain forest north of the river. But only in 1875 was a serious expedition mounted by Count Brazza, an Italian who represented French interests. Ascending the river, he decided it was not a good way into the rain forest and headed south toward the Congo River. He was obstructed by local people at the banks of the Alima but in 1880 finally reached the Congo at what is now Brazzaville, near Kinshasa.

The rain forest north of the Ogooué remained unmapped by outsiders until 1895, when the explorer Mary Kingsley started her expedition. Accompanied by a servant, this thirty-three-year-old daughter of an English doctor ascended the Ogooué River along the same track as Brazza. However, where Brazza had turned south, she bravely turned north and eventually planted her visiting card at the top of Mount Cameroon. As such explorations of the western equatorial rain forest increased, HIV-0 could begin to leave its isolation.

But if chimpanzees gave us their virus, where did they get it? If both chimpanzees and humans got the virus from the same third animal, what was it? The Zairian SIV cpz-ant is the virus closest to both the SIV cpz-gab/HIV-1 cluster and the SIV cpz-us/HIV-0 cluster. Its genetic distance from both clusters suggests that SIV cpz has circulated for hundreds to thousands of years among chimpanzees. Apparently, in one troop of apes, SIV cpz-ant evolved into a virus close to HIV-1; in another troop, it evolved into a virus closer to HIV-0. Yet despite centuries of ape-to-ape passages,

SIV cpz has never gained the ability to cause AIDS in these animals, except possibly under rare experimental conditions. In contrast, its descendant became lethal in humans after a much shorter period of circulation.

Perhaps SIV once caused AIDS in chimpanzees but is now attenuated, or weakened, in virulence. In any case, chimpanzees have been much luckier than we have. Whether infected with SIV in the wild or in the laboratory, chimpanzees have a very low virus load. Their minimal level of virus production is seen only in the few humans designated nonprogressors. Constituting less than 1 percent of all people infected with HIV-1, these long-term asymptomatic survivors seem to share a genetic constitution that is rare in the general population. Their virus load is so feeble that their immune system is unfazed, and they are not very infectious to other people. The same is probably true for the chimpanzees, who show no detrimental effects of infection (by SIV cpz or by HIV-1) and appear to spread their virus very slowly.

SIV cpz has been found in only four animals, partly because chimpanzees are not susceptible until sexually active but also, no doubt, because SIV cpz virus load and spread are so low compared with HIV and SIV in other monkeys. If ape-to-ape transmission is so rare, then ape-to-human transmission must be even rarer, unless humans are more vulnerable than chimpanzees themselves—not an easy hypothesis to test!

The extremely low virus load in chimpanzees makes them increasingly suspect as our direct source of HIV-1 or HIV-0. In any case, chimpanzees most likely got their virus the same way we did: by hunting and eating their primate relatives. When their hunting behavior was studied in the rain forests of Ivory Coast and Tanzania, they were found to eat several kinds of deer, but mostly monkeys. About three-quarters of their prey consisted of monkeys, about half of them full-grown and thus able to carry SIV. Adolescent and adult male chimpanzees do most of the hunting but share the kill with females of the troop. So in addition to their usual fruit, both males and females eat baboons, sooty mangabeys, and guenons like redtail monkeys and diana monkeys.

But their favorite food, by far, is the red colobus monkey, also a favorite of local humans. A colobus SIV has not yet been isolated but could well be the true ancestor of HIV-0 and HIV-1.

6

HIV-2: The Sooty Mangabey Connection

In September of 1984, the year that HIV-1 was unmistakably identified as the prime cause of AIDS, a similar virus was isolated from Asian monkeys by Ron Desrosiers at Harvard's New England Primate Center in Massachusetts. These research animals had an AIDS-like disease, as did Asian monkeys at several other US primate facilities. None had been infected in the wild. The Harvard animals had been infected by four rhesus macaques shipped in 1970 from the California Regional Primate Center, where they were exposed in the 1960s to sooty mangabeys. On testing, the sootys proved to be SIV-positive.

This epidemic among captive primates affected only Asian monkeys, not African monkeys. The AIDS-like immunodeficiency developed over about 10 years, and SIV infection was invariably traced to housing of Asian monkeys with sooty mangabeys or injection with their blood or tissues. The new viruses were called SIV mac and SIV stm since they were isolated from diseased rhesus macaques and stump-tailed macaques. Apparently Asian monkeys, like humans, could get AIDS after infection with viruses that in their natural hosts cause no disease. Sooty mangabeys are often infected with SIV sm but without harm. In contrast, Asian monkeys never encounter SIV in the wild but, when infected, become deathly ill.

To investigate the AIDS potential of the usually innocent SIV sm, studies were performed at various institutions. In our own studies at the Dutch Primate Center, we first infected ten rhesus monkeys from India with SIV isolated from a sooty mangabey. All but one rhesus got AIDS an average of two years after inoculation. The disease looked very much like AIDS in humans: the monkeys developed *P. carinii* pneumonia (PCP) that was often combined with a generalized cytomegalovirus (CMV) infection. White blood cells from one of the nine diseased monkeys were injected into another rhesus, who developed AIDS in less than a year. His cells were injected into a rhesus who developed AIDS in less than half a year. Then blood cells were taken from this animal and injected into four others. All developed AIDS in under three months. When we repeated this process two more times, AIDS developed in a month.

This experiment provides three very important insights. It confirms that a virus of the SIV/HIV family that does not cause AIDS in its natural host (in this case, the sooty mangabey) may be quite deadly in a susceptible host that has never encountered SIV in the wild. What we saw with Asian monkeys in captivity could well have happened to humans in Africa, as we will show later.

It also shows that the symptom-free period can vary in individuals (in this case, Asian monkeys), even when they receive exactly the same amount of the same virus at exactly the same time. Of our first ten animals, two developed AIDS as soon as seven months after injection, and two others developed AIDS as long as three years after injection. This demonstrates the importance of host factors in setting the course of infection. It explains why some people develop AIDS in a few months while others show no signs even after decades of infection.

Finally, this experiment confirms that rapid passage in a new species can increase virulence. SIV from the sooty mangabey became reproducibly more aggressive upon every new monkey-to-monkey passage of blood cells. This is no doubt what happened to HIV-1 in the Lake Victoria area when, in the 1970s, it gained new opportunity from the sexual activities of traders and soldiers.

The SIV from sooty mangabeys clearly has AIDS potential when it meets a previously unexposed species of primates. But is it likely to meet such victims in the wild? Sootys live in rain forest west of the Dahomey

Gap, ranging from West African Guinea and Sierra Leone to Ivory Coast. In 1992, blood was collected from twenty-two free-ranging sootys from Sierra Leone by Preston Marx, a virologist at the Aaron Diamond Research Center in New York. He tested ten animals, a random sample, and found four infected with SIV sm. He isolated one of the viruses, which turned out to be the most divergent SIV found to date. This isolate apparently represented a group of sooty viruses that had started both the HIV-2 epidemic and the SIV epidemic among captive macaques, since it was genetically equidistant from HIV-2 and SIV mac.

Meanwhile, van der Groen and Piot looked for SIV among assorted Ivory Coast monkeys. They tested six baboons, twenty-eight African green monkeys, six sooty mangabeys, and three patas monkeys for antibodies to HIV-2, which we know is closely related to SIV sm. They found four monkeys positive: one of the African green monkeys, and three of the six sootys. They isolated virus from two of the three sootys, one of which had been captured in 1979, the other in 1991. Both animals came from villages in the rain forest of Ivory Coast close to the Liberian border. Their viruses were, like the Marx isolate, very close to the SIVs isolated previously from animals at US primate centers.

The American and Belgian studies yielded small numbers but show that SIV is endemic among sootys after they reach sexual maturity. (Monkeys in the wild appear to be SIV-infected almost exclusively by the sexual route.) The studies confirmed suspicions that SIV sm, the same virus that caused AIDS in captive Asian monkeys, indeed circulates in the wild. Though harmless in African monkeys and therefore unnoticed, it is deadly to primates unaccustomed to it, including humans. Since African peoples hunt monkeys for food and commonly keep sootys as pets, SIV sm has plenty of opportunity to infect and pass among these humans. Unlike SIV cpz, its cross-species transmission to humans—now, and for centuries past—is not a rare fluke but an everyday event.

Soon after SIV sm was linked to AIDS among rhesus monkeys, it was linked to AIDS among humans in West Africa. In 1984 a group in Dakar, Senegal, found the first clue. The group was headed by Souleyman M'Boup, a physician who studies and treats sexually transmitted disease. He had noticed among his patients a high incidence of Burkitt's lymphoma, a tumor caused by a herpesvirus related to the one that causes Kaposi's sarcoma (KS). Others had already noticed that this lymphoma occurs in people with AIDS risk factors such as sexually transmitted disease. But when M'Boup tested his patients for antibodies to HIV-1, he got negative or equivocal results. He subsequently gave samples to Francis Barin, a French virologist on his way to the laboratory of Max Essex, an expert on retroviruses at Harvard's School of Public Health.

The prostitutes who gave the samples were not ill. However, they belonged to the same high-risk group in which M'Boup had noticed the Burkitt's lymphoma and other opportunistic infections in the absence of HIV-1. At the Essex lab, Barin found that many of these women were infected with a virus that cross-reacted with the SIV isolated from captive rhesus macaques. This finding immediately proved two things. Beside HIV-1 and HIV-0, another virus of the same family was causing AIDS; and not only chimpanzee viruses threatened humans but also viruses from monkeys like the sooty mangabey (which had infected the macaques).

Montagnier decided to attempt isolation of the mysterious new virus. In October 1985 he received promising samples from Portuguese virologist Marie-Odette Santos-Ferreira. She had obtained them from an HIV-1 negative AIDS patient from Guinea-Bissau (a former Portuguese colony in West Africa) under treatment at Lisbon's Egas Moniz Hospital. As mentioned in Chapter 3, Montagnier's group soon recovered the new virus and named it HIV-2. Their work made it possible to produce reagents for specific detection of HIV-2 infections in West Africa and the rest of the world.

HIV-2 was found to be almost exclusively restricted to West Africa, the habitat of sooty mangabeys and SIV sm. The prostitutes of West African coastal towns, from Senegal to Nigeria, are its population of highest prevalence. In most of West Africa, its infections could have come directly from sootys but, since these monkeys do not cross the Dahomey Gap, infections in Nigeria must have been spread human-to-human. The few HIV-2 infections outside of West Africa are found in European countries with former colonial ties, such as Portugal and France. Infections are seen mostly among people who have come to these European countries directly from West African areas where HIV-2 is endemic.

HIV-2, like HIV-0 and HIV-1, can only have arisen in Africa. Like HIV-0, it was discovered to cause AIDS only after HIV-1 launched the AIDS epidemic and antibody testing was developed. Whether HIV-0 is weak or strong is still a question, but HIV-2 is, without doubt, the weakest of all AIDS viruses. It spreads very slowly; it causes AIDS very infrequently and after a long asymptomatic period. In many years of watching and waiting, we have seen only a small percentage of people progress to AIDS after infection with HIV-2. This is quite amazing for a virus that belongs to the same family as the deadly HIV-1. In most of its human hosts, HIV-2 produces extremely little virus. In HIV-1 hosts, such minimal production and virus load is seen only in the very few and fortunate nonprogressors.

The HIV-2 epidemic is as slow as the virus. No evidence hints that HIV-2 caused AIDS at any location in Africa before HIV-1 emerged in the 1970s. The first confirmed case of AIDS caused by HIV-2 occurred in 1978, at least ten years after the Norwegian sailor was infected with HIV-0 and two years after the first African HIV-1 isolate was obtained. Clearly HIV-2 was late to cause AIDS, but we cannot tell whether it was transmitted to humans before or after HIV-1 and HIV-0. We suspect a long history of passage but have no evidence because the low transmissibility and low profile of HIV-2 make its infections very hard to spot. Much time and effort are needed to detect the rare AIDS case caused by this elusive member of the HIV family.

The first confirmed case of AIDS caused by HIV-2 concerned a forty-three-year-old man, living in Portugal, who was referred to the Hospital for Tropical Diseases in London. For two years he had suffered intermittent fever, diarrhea, weight loss, and abdominal pain. He had lived in Guinea-Bissau from 1956 to 1966. Presumably, the virus found him during that time. If so, in the rare cases in which HIV-2 causes AIDS, it may progress about as fast as HIV-1, which causes AIDS in an average of ten years. By 1978 this man had severe wasting disease, an abnormally low CD4+ cell count, and a documented cryptosporidium infection. Cryptosporidium is an intestinal parasite that rarely causes disease in humans unless they are immunocompromised. All these clinical and immunological signs are diagnostic of AIDS. After three months of treatment in the United Kingdom, the man continued to suffer from severe diarrhea, and he returned to Portugal to die.

Sera were collected three times from this patient during 1978. Each time, testing for HIV-1 antibodies gave results that were officially negative but showed some reactivity to HIV-1 core proteins. This semipositive result could mean absolutely nothing. Like most tests, the test for HIV-1 occasionally gives a false-positive result. But the result could also mean that the patient had a very early HIV-1 infection—or was infected by a virus related to HIV-1. When HIV-2 testing became available, this man's sera reacted well with coat proteins of HIV-2, as did sera from his wife. So his case is considered the first documented HIV-2 infection to have AIDS as the clinical result.

As soon as HIV-2 was identified in 1985, it began to look like a virus acquired by direct monkey-to-human transmission. Whereas HIV-1 and HIV-0 strains were far removed from SIV cpz, HIV-2 strains were only a few generations—perhaps just a single generation—removed from SIV sm. This was clear from their close resemblance to the SIV of diseased rhesus macaques, who had acquired their virus directly from sootys mangabeys. Humans might easily acquire a virus directly from sootys since Africans share the sooty habitat and keep sootys as pets.

So the search was on for a true monkey virus in a human host, that is, a first-generation HIV-2, transmitted directly from a monkey to its first human. Nobody has yet looked systematically in the most logical place, among forest people, but Beatrice Hahn has come close. Her Alabama group collected sera from Liberian adults living in three areas: the capital of Monrovia, a rubber plantation in central Liberia, and isolated rain forest villages in the north. In the Monrovian sample the researchers found three HIV infections (including one case of frank AIDS), all HIV-1. In the rural samples they found five HIV infections (no AIDS), all HIV-2.

This distribution shows clearly how HIV-1 and HIV-2 have entered the population of West Africa. HIV-1 emerged first in the urban areas, reaching its highest prevalence among prostitutes. In 1986 about 20 percent of prostitutes in Abidjan, the capital of Ivory Coast, were infected with HIV-1. By 1990 that percentage had at least doubled. Among the same prostitutes, fewer than 10 percent were infected with HIV-2 in 1986, and their number had declined by 1990. These facts from a second West African capital strongly suggest that HIV-1 not only spread rapidly in the big cities but very likely originated there. Unfortunately, we have no documentation as to how or when it came to West Africa. The subtype we see there is mainly HIV-1A, which has its epicenter in East Africa, especially Rwanda. Instead of coming by the truck routes, HIV-1A seems to have jumped from east to west by air travel between French-speaking countries (see Figure 4.4).

In contrast to HIV-1, HIV-2 does not seem to have spread after having reached the capitals of West Africa. It is as if the virus made its appearance and thereafter could not sustain itself very effectively in the urban population. This is not surprising, since HIV-2 spreads poorly. The surprise is that it survives at all in urban areas, competing with HIV-1. Two explanations come to mind. First, individuals with HIV-2 infection remain healthy long enough to reach the threshold number of sexual encounters needed to pass on the virus. Second, the HIV-2 circulating in cities is continually replenished by new strains acquired rurally by monkey-to-human transmission. Unlike HIV-1, which has traveled far to invade West African cities, HIV-2 comes from villages only a bus ride away.

Sampling in remote areas of West Africa finds that of one hundred people, one to five are infected with HIV-2. Their strains show surprising variation. Comparable variation in HIV-1 is easily explained by the relatively long history of the virus and its rapid human-to-human transmission. What explains such variation in slow-spreading HIV-2? One might postulate that, whereas HIV-1 variation stems from a few ape-to-human transmissions followed by long human circulation, the myriad variants of HIV-2 stem from many everyday monkey-to-human transmissions followed by relatively little human circulation. This pattern seems likely since many sootys have SIV, and many live close to humans. The virus would spread in blood or saliva, most often the latter. Pet sootys are rarely eaten but may bite if teased. They often turn snappish with age.

Final evidence for the direct monkey origin of HIV-2 came from genetic analysis of viruses from two of Hahn's five rural Liberians, both rubber workers in good health. As explained in Chapter 3, the best way to analyze relationships between two or more viruses is to study a stretch of nucleic acids from a gene or gene fragment they have in common. Such shared genes have the same function and general configuration but may vary in nucleic acid detail. The more details that differ from one virus to another, the more distantly related the viruses. Hahn used this technique to compare the two Liberian HIV-2 viruses with SIVs from captive sootys, SIVs from captive rhesus macaques infected by sootys, and, most important, SIV from a pet sooty wild-caught in Liberia. She also compared the two rubber workers' HIV-2 strains to all known HIV-2 strains.

As might be expected, Hahn confirmed that HIV-2 and SIV strains from sooty mangabeys and infected rhesus macaques form one big family, which is only very distantly related to HIV-1, HIV-0, and the chimpanzee viruses. Clearly, the human, ape, and monkey viruses of the lentivirus family do not cluster according to species. HIV-2 of humans is far closer to the SIV of sooty mangabeys than to HIV-1 or HIV-0, or to the chimpanzee viruses. Conversely, human HIV-0 and HIV-1 are closely related to the chimpanzee viruses but only distant cousins of HIV-2.

This lack of clustering by species proves that HIV-0, HIV-1, and HIV-2 lack a common human virus ancestor. Likewise, viruses like SIV sm and SIV cpz have no common nonhuman primate virus ancestor. HIV-0 and

HIV-1 are the result of chimpanzee-to-human transmission and therefore share a common ancestor. HIV-2, the result of sooty-to-human transmission, has a common ancestor with SIV sm.

When Hahn performed her analysis, a family tree of HIV-2 and SIV sm strains had already been drawn. The HIV-2 strains formed two main branches, while the SIVs formed a third. Genetic analysis of HIV-2 and SIV strains had strongly suggested a direct relationship, but proof was lacking until Hahn analyzed the HIV-2 strains of the two rubber workers. One of these, designated HIV-2$_{2238}$, fit on one of the two HIV-2 branches and thus revealed nothing new, but the other provided the missing link. This virus, HIV-2$_{F0784}$, adjoined the SIV branch. It was the most SIV-like of HIV-2 strains. In fact, it was much more closely related to SIVs from sootys and rhesus monkeys than to any HIV-2 strains. It was, at last, a true monkey virus: an SIV lately transmitted to its first human, a first-generation HIV-2 just adapting to its new host species. Its immediate ancestor was not another HIV-2 but the very same kind of SIV that Marx had found among free-ranging sootys in Sierra Leone.

Of course, a skeptic could argue that transmission went the other way. Hahn's missing link could point to "the first human viruses seen in monkeys." However, it seems unlikely that a human virus from Liberia could simultaneously infect sootys in several parts of West Africa and macaques in the United States. How could a plantation worker, who never left Liberia, infect macaques who went from Asia to the United States without ever stopping in Liberia? Besides, HIV-2$_{F0784}$ and SIV mac seem equidistantly descended from SIV sm but much closer to each other than to their parent. So the best bet is that the worker in Liberia and the macaques in the United States were infected by SIV sm at about the same time. The resulting first generation of both HIV-2 and SIV mac/stm therefore evolved about the same distance from SIV sm (though somewhat differently) to set up housekeeping in their new hosts. And since neither host, man or macaque, had previously encountered SIV, both developed AIDS.

If HIV-2 comes from monkeys with long and frequent human contact, how long has it caused human disease? What was this virus doing before its "discovery" in 1985? Since SIV sm never makes sootys sick, they must have carried it for many generations, even millennia. (The common ancestor of the SIV and HIV lineage—the root of the SIV/HIV tree—is thought to go back hundreds and perhaps thousands of years.) In all that time, sootys surely had many opportunities to infect people. Transmission of SIV sm to humans must have been very common. It seems astonishing that we only now recognize the deadly effect of this virus on humans.

On second thought, there are good reasons. HIV-2 went unnoticed among the isolated forest people because of its slow spread and low disease potential. When a person finally showed signs of HIV-2 infection, the illness might be laid to one of many causes, natural or supernatural. A case of AIDS would hardly be noticed among the other fatal diseases that have plagued Africans for centuries. Also, many potential victims would die from other causes—disease, injury, or the harsh conditions of life—long before their HIV-2 infection could progress to AIDS.

Beyond the forest people, HIV-2 went unnoticed until forest areas began to be cultivated and Europeans came during the nineteenth century. Once timber trade opened trade routes, the forest people were less isolated. But even in this century, as forest people have trickled into urban areas, HIV-2 remained hidden because of its slow and subtle course of infection. Its rare cases of AIDS could not be spotted until eyes were opened to the phenomenon of virus-induced immunodeficiency. This awareness came after HIV-1 had caused numerous cases of AIDS. Only after the HIV-1 epidemic started and AIDS testing was developed could anyone recognize AIDS caused by another more subtle virus.

The Sabaeus Connection

If sooty mangabeys have carried SIV for thousands of years, where did they get this ancestor to HIV-2? Nothing close to SIV sm has been found in species other than sootys and humans. However, isolated genes or gene fragments of SIV sm are found in the SIV of an even smaller monkey, the sabaeus monkey, a subspecies of African green monkey. This SIV agm with sooty virus genes is, of course, the recombinant of a parent SIV agm and a parent SIV sm.

African green monkeys (*Cercopithecus aethiops*) are a species of guenon. Native to Africa, they live only on that continent, except for some that were introduced to the West Indies in the seventeenth century. African green monkeys are one of the most successful primates of Africa, probably because they are small and thrive in trees or on the ground, eating whatever is handy. They reproduce rapidly in almost any habitat that offers a few trees, some water, and minimal variation in food.

Four subspecies of African green monkeys are generally recognized. They include sabaeus or green monkeys (*Cercopithecus aethiops sabaeus*), tantalus monkeys (*C. a. tantalus*), grivets (*C. a. aethiops*), and vervets (*C. a. pygerythrus*). These subspecies do not form very stable genetic clusters, although the sabaeus monkeys are the most stable of the lot. The four subspecies are often seen as one species with four populations divided geographically by their habitats. The sabaeus population typically stays within West Africa, ranging from about the savanna of Senegal in the west to the Volta River in the east—roughly the same range as sootys. Tantalus monkeys inhabit the sub-Saharan region from about the Volta to the Nile. They also inhabit Zaire north of the Congo River, and the northwestern part of Uganda. Grivets live in the region extending from the Sudan (east of the Nile and south of Khartoum) into Ethiopia except for the south of that country. Vervets live in southern Ethiopia and Somalia, South Africa, and also Uganda, eastern Zaire, and Zambia east of the Luangwa River (Figures 6.1 and 6.2).

As far as we know, African green monkeys are the species of monkey most commonly infected with SIV. More are infected than sootys, for example, but like sootys they suffer no ill effects. Up to 50 percent of African green monkeys are infected once past reproductive age. Each of the four subspecies has its own brand of SIV, but all are called SIV agm. Of the four, the sabaeus SIV agm is the only recombinant. This and other evidence suggests that vervets, grivets, and tantalus monkeys each had a well-established SIV agm before the sabaeus monkeys did. Perhaps SIV agm spread east to west in its species population, reaching West Africa last. In any case, it appears that sabaeus monkeys had no well-established SIV. At some point, two candidates arose in the population: the parents of the recombinant SIV agm they carry today. One parent was a vervet, grivet, or tantalus SIV agm. The other was the future SIV sm, ancestor of HIV-2. Apparently unsuccessful among the sabaeus (compared with its recombinant offspring), it would be more successful in the neighboring sooty population.

The Hahn group has discovered some important features of the recombinant SIV of sabaeus monkeys. Any SIV or HIV genome, when spliced into the genome of the host cell, has a binding site for the so-called *tat* protein. Essential for efficient virus reproduction, this site, called *tar*, is present in a single copy in vervet, grivet, and tantalus SIVs. It is duplicated in

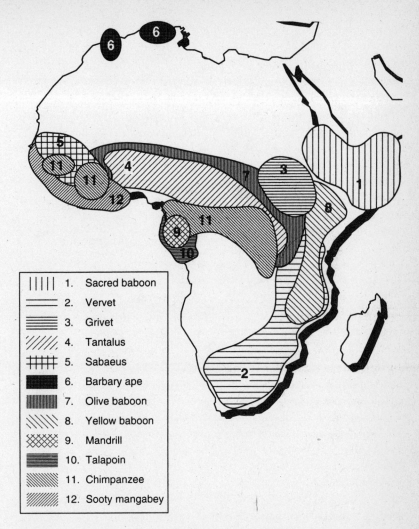

Figure 6.1 **Distribution in Africa of major nonhuman primate species**.
*Most relevant to our story are the African green monkey, particularly the sabaeus
subspecies, the sooty mangabey, Barbary ape, talapoin, chimpanzee, and various
baboons. Also relevant are the colobus monkeys, a minor population that shares
habitat with chimpanzees. (Haltenorth 1977.)*

Legend:

1. Sacred baboon
2. Vervet
3. Grivet
4. Tantalus
5. Sabaeus
6. Barbary ape
7. Olive baboon
8. Yellow baboon
9. Mandrill
10. Talapoin
11. Chimpanzee
12. Sooty mangabey

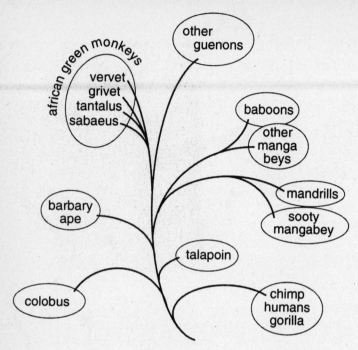

Figure 6.2 The family tree of African human and nonhuman primates.
Based on genetic evidence, mandrills are closely related to sooty mangabeys, whereas other mangabeys are closer to baboons. Talapoins appear to be a completely separate species, as do Barbary apes. The Barbary ape is most closely related to Asian macaques and may be their ancestor. (van der Kuyl et al. 1995.)

the sabaeus SIV agm, however, and also in SIV sm and HIV-2. In most other ways the sabaeus SIV agm is just like the SIV agm of vervets, grivets, and tantalus monkeys. But unlike them, its genome has genes and gene fragments in common with SIV sm and HIV-2. This "mosaic," or mixed, genome has been found in enough sabaeus SIVs to suggest that it is a characteristic feature.

Only viral sex can explain the mosaic structure of the sabaeus virus, yet the recombinant result is very surprising. Remember that many humans in

West Africa have been found with a double infection of HIV-1 and HIV-2. Yet never, to date, have these viruses created a recombinant. These two HIV species may not infect the same cells of the body with equal efficiency. More likely, they lack sufficient overlap to produce progeny, or their progeny lacks any survival advantage and is immediately outcompeted by the parents and other strains. We can assume that viruses as genetically different as HIV-1 and HIV-2 are virtually unable to form a recombinant that can survive and multiply. Since the parents of the sabaeus recombinant were genetically different to about the same extent, how could they accomplish this feat? (More about this later.) In any case, it appears that sabaeus monkeys gave their cast-off virus to sooty mangabeys, who gave it to us.

While the subspecies of African green monkey do not form clear or stable genetic clusters, their viruses do. Vervet viruses always cluster with other vervet viruses, grivet viruses with grivet viruses, and so on. This viral clustering suggests that the host subspecies and their SIVs have coevolved. Each virus has evolved on the shirttails of the monkey it inhabits, following the changes of its host. But this makes sense only if the genome of each monkey subspecies is mirrored by the genome of its particular SIV. Hahn showed this is not the case for the green monkey and its mosaic SIV.

Some scientists believe that monkeys and their respective SIVs have coevolved for millions of years, but the evidence can be read another way. Since the African green monkey subspecies do not cluster clearly, the clustering of their viruses could actually argue against coevolution. Instead, the viral clusters could result from the long and strict geographic separation of the monkey subspecies. After all, coevolution cannot explain the sabaeus SIV, the stable recombinant of SIV sm and SIV from a vervet, grivet, or tantalus monkey. (Obviously, the sabaeus monkeys who host the recombinant are not, themselves, recombinants of a sooty mangabey and a vervet, grivet, or tantalus monkey.) Studies have shown that the viruses of South African vervets cluster separately from those of East African vervets. These two clusters of vervet viruses are part of the same close-knit family although their host populations are a thousand miles apart. Meanwhile, viruses of grivets and tantalus monkeys, whose hosts live close together, belong to two clearly separate families. The best nongenetic explanation is that the tantalus and grivet ranges are more sharply divided geographically than the two vervet ranges.

Clues From the Caribbean

To put the coevolution theory completely to rest, we need to find sabaeus monkeys that still carry the SIV that was evicted by the recombinant SIV agm. We need to find the parent that moved into sootys as SIV sm, then passed to humans. How can we find this virus, the ancestor of HIV-2? We see its remnants in the sabaeus recombinant, but it apparently has disappeared from sabaeus monkeys in Africa. We need a sabaeus population whose ancestors left Africa before the recombination event. The ancestors must have been sufficiently numerous to include a few SIV-infected monkeys. The descendant population must, ever since, have remained completely separate from sabaeus monkeys in Africa, so their original SIV (if present) could thrive without competition from the recombinant. Such complete separation usually requires more than distance. It requires an environmental barrier such as sharp climatic change or a large body of water.

The perfect population may exist in the Caribbean. The rain forests of St. Kitts, Nevis, and Barbados are full of sabaeus monkeys whose ancestors were imported from Africa as long as 350 years ago. We do not yet know if the ancestors left Africa before the recombination event, but they could have. We do not yet know if their descendants are infected with SIV—original or recombinant—but their history makes them worth testing as we search for the ancestor of HIV-2.

Their importation seems to have started at St. Kitts and spread soon to nearby Nevis. The British established St. Kitts and Nevis as colonies in 1623 and 1628, respectively, but from 1627 to 1665 the French held land on both tips of St. Kitts. In 1665 the rival powers declared war, and the twin islands went back and forth until the British finally secured them in 1713. Either the British or the French could have imported sabaeus monkeys from Africa, but only the French are mentioned in reports we have found. For example, a report from 1700 mentions pet monkeys escaping from French homes on St. Kitts, presumably during a British attack on a French enclave. An earlier report tells of a seventeenth-century shipment—330 monkeys in boxes and cages—transported from French holdings in West Africa to buyers in France.

One can assume that these monkeys, exported from French West African colonies to France or other colonies, were sabaeus monkeys since West Africa is the exclusive habitat of this subspecies. Indeed, the monkeys I have seen on St. Kitts clearly resemble sabaeus or green monkeys from

West Africa, with their green-gold back, a yellowish white front, and a black face bordered by white hair. Genetic analysis in our laboratory has recently confirmed their West African origin.

The monkeys on Barbados offer an independent population to test for the original sabaeus SIV agm. I have not seen these monkeys but doubt that they come from St. Kitts and Nevis, which are too far from Barbados. Nor are the monkeys likely to have come from French West Africa, since the French never had a presence on Barbados. Only the British colonized this island, which was their main West Indian port. Apparently, it was inhabited only by New World monkeys (most likely *Cebus capucinus*) until the mid–nineteenth century, when Old World monkeys began to be imported. They were probably from St. Jago and other Cape Verdean Islands, a sabaeus habitat, because since the seventeenth century the British had captured those monkeys there. The so-called St. Jago monkey was once a fashionable pet in England. It was also the type specimen Linnaeus used in 1766 to distinguish sabaeus or green monkeys as a taxonomic entity.

Sufficient documentation exists to suggest that two distinct sabaeus populations left Africa for the West Indies. The oldest population, on St. Kitts and Nevis, most likely came between 1627 and 1713 from French settlements in Senegal and the Gambia. Over those eighty-six years, French ships must have sailed often between Africa and the West Indies. Many ships must have carried monkeys, which were popular with sailors as pets or mascots. Many monkeys must have jumped ship and ended up living on the islands. At a conservative estimate, ten trips per year, each adding just one sabaeus monkey to the island population, would in eighty-six years bring that population to 860. This number would surely include a few SIV-infected adults who would circulate the virus. If it was the original sabaeus SIV agm, which in Africa became SIV sm, the chances are good that this virus can be isolated among the estimated 45,000 sabaeus monkeys on St. Kitts today.

The chances are not so good on Barbados, where a much smaller sabaeus population was established much later, over a shorter period of importation. Its ancestors may have been too few to include any SIV-infected monkeys. If ancestors were infected, they are more likely than the St. Kitts and Nevis monkeys to have brought the recombinant SIV agm, not the original virus, since they left Africa just 150 years ago.

Still, they are worth testing. Hendry (1986) reported that ninety-eight Caribbean green monkeys, bled from 1980 to 1985, were all negative for SIV from captive macaques. However, those green monkeys were unidentified as to age or locale. Perhaps they were too young to be SIV-infected; perhaps they were from Barbados. We can still hope that someone will test adult sabaeus monkeys from St. Kitts and Nevis, and find the lost SIV.

Meanwhile, back in Africa, no SIV agm has caused disease in its natural host, whether vervet, grivet, tantalus, or sabaeus monkey. However, like SIV sm, it can cause disease in a species of Asian monkeys: the pig-tailed macaque. This means that, given the right circumstances, SIV agm is a killer virus like SIV sm. Especially since sootys and sabaeus monkeys share habitat, the original SIV agm might easily have infected a sooty and started a chain of infections leading to HIV-2. One way to learn more is to study the virus of sabaeus monkeys that share trees with sooty mangabeys.

The question remains how or why two SIVs achieved the feat of recombination, when even HIV-0 and HIV-1 have not. An answer could be that a survival advantage accrued to the monkey viruses but not to the human viruses, as explained in Chapter 3. Unfortunately we cannot prove this. We cannot demonstrate, for example, that the recombinant SIV agm spreads more efficiently in sabaeus monkey blood cells than did the parent SIVs. But the most important survival advantage for a poorly transmissible virus is to enhance its potential to transmit, so perhaps this explains the recombinant.

In any case, this anomaly serves us by linking SIV sm (and therefore HIV-2) with SIVs from vervets, grivets, and tantalus monkeys through their hosts. Once the recombinant SIV agm appeared, a battle for survival ensued as the new virus competed with the old one in the sabaeus population. We do not know why the recombinant triumphed (perhaps it spread faster or was less lethal to its host), but it did. The old virus gradually disappeared from sabaeus monkeys but found a home with sooty mangabeys, thus becoming the ancestor of SIV sm and HIV-2.

The Baboon Connection

Recent evidence suggests that a vervet SIV has infected baboons. To understand this, it helps to look at the family tree of all African monkeys and apes. In 1995, when we sequenced part of the monkey genomes, we showed that this tree has four main branches plus talapoins, discussed in Chapter 10. As shown in Figure 6.2, these four represent humans and great apes; red colobus and other colobines; guenons, notably the African green monkeys; and the Papionini tribe. This tribe can be seen as three main groups: mandrills and sooty mangabeys; black mangabeys, tana mangabeys, and olive and chacma baboons; and Barbary apes or *Macaca sylvana*, the only macaque living in Africa. No SIV has been found in Barbary apes. SIVs have been found in both mandrills and sooty mangabeys, but they represent two distinct virus families that preclude coevolution of viruses with hosts. Black mangabeys and tana mangabeys have not been found to harbor any SIV. However, rare infections have been found in baboons. (Note that mandrills, a type of baboon, are grouped apart from other baboon species. Their viral susceptibility pattern differs, and whenever this book refers to baboons without designating species, the reader can assume mandrills are excluded.)

Based on their features, baboons are divided into yellow, olive, sacred, and chacma types. Our analysis, in line with many others, found the first three to be genetically identical; the fourth differs only slightly from the others. SIV infections were first found in these animals in 1989. At that time Desrosiers of the New England Primate Center tested two groups for antibodies to SIV sm and SIV agm: 123 yellow baboons of the Mikumi National Park in central Tanzania, and 119 olive and sacred baboons of the Awash National Park in Ethiopia. Two yellow baboons from Tanzania were seropositive, and none of the Ethiopian baboons. But since yellow, olive, and sacred baboons are genetically alike, we must suspect that all three groups are susceptible, if not also the chacma. Antibodies from the two seropositive baboons reacted more vigorously with SIV agm than with SIV sm, suggesting infection with a virus closely related to African green monkey viruses. Both seropositive animals were adult females from a troop of 34, of which 21 were tested. The Desrosiers group noticed African green monkeys, most likely vervets, living close by this troop. They suspected that the two females had been infected by vervets, especially since baboons eat African green monkeys (albeit much less often than chimpanzees eat colobus monkeys).

Since SIV agm viruses cluster according to their host, genetic analysis could tell whether the two baboons were infected by a vervet SIV or some other SIV agm. Again, Beatrice Hahn tackled the problem. Desrosiers supplied DNA from the two SIV-infected baboons, and Hahn managed to recover SIV gene fragments from one of these animals. They were identified as part of an East African vervet virus, so Desrosiers had guessed right: this baboon was indeed infected by a vervet.

Hahn subsequently looked at the evolutionary characteristics of the vervet virus in baboons compared with the virus in its natural vervet host. When a virus enters an unaccustomed host and starts to produce disease, the viral DNA suddenly changes to make new proteins. Such changes have been seen with transmission of SIV to humans and Asian monkeys, and they were seen with transmission of the vervet SIV to baboons. The type and number of changes told Hahn that baboons are relatively new SIV hosts, as are humans and Asian monkeys. Unlike the chimpanzee, mandrill, sooty mangabey, and the four types of African green monkey, the baboon seems to be the first African primate host to be recently infected. Unlike the others, it has not been infected long enough for the host-virus accommodation or equilibrium that prevents disease.

Does SIV agm cause disease in baboons? We cannot be sure because data are still so sparse. We only know, from the Desrosiers studies, that even after reproductive age, adult baboons are seldom SIV-infected in the wild. Perhaps these animals are only barely susceptible to SIV agm, making transmission a rare and transient event. No one has yet tried to infect baboons with SIV agm in the laboratory. However, some baboons have developed an AIDS-like illness after experimental infection with HIV-2, which suggests they are in the same category as humans and Asian monkeys. They are apparently susceptible not only to SIV/HIV infection but also to development of life-threatening disease due to virus-induced immunodeficiency.

To sum up, an SIV agm long ago infected sabaeus monkeys, and more recently infected baboons. Sabaeus monkeys passed their virus to sooty mangabeys, which passed it to humans and rhesus monkeys, which both got AIDS from the sooty virus. The history of HIV-2 strongly suggests that AIDS is a zoonosis, a disease originating from an animal—in this case, a nonhuman primate. Without doubt, African green monkeys have carried SIV for millennia. Sootys and mandrills also have carried SIV a long time. By now they are infected without harm, but perhaps when SIV first entered these populations, it caused disease.

SIVs have not become attenuated in their ability to spread. They appear to have become attenuated in their ability to cause disease—but how can we tell? We must compare today's innocent strains with presumably less innocent strains that circulated a few thousand years ago. Luckily, we have an ingenious vehicle for this molecular time travel.

7

Searching for SIV
in Monkey Mummies

To trace genetic changes that could have made SIV into a harmless virus of African green monkeys and sooty mangabeys, we needed to find SIV in an ancient and possibly harmful form. How can we do this?

When SIV infects white blood cells, its RNA converts to DNA and moves into the host cell genome. There it stays—harmless or not—for the life of the host, and sometimes in postmortem remains. Since SIV infects monkeys at reproductive age, its presence in host cells should persist as the animal ages, reaching a high level by the end of a typical life span. So our best chance to find ancient SIV was to find SIV-infected adult monkeys that died in ancient times but retained tissue that might contain white blood cells. In the DNA of such monkey cells we might find some integrated stretches of SIV DNA.

As this chapter will tell, monkey mummies twenty-five hundred to five thousand years old can be found and studied. Techniques exist to recover SIV DNA from the DNA of ancient monkeys, to amplify the viral material in the test tube, and to analyze its virulence and other characteristics. But before one can study ancient SIV DNA, one must find the right monkeys:

those likely to be SIV-infected. One must find tissue containing blood cell remains. One must find the nearly vanished traces of SIV DNA buried in the ancient monkey DNA. Above all, one must make sure the ancient monkey DNA is truly monkey and truly ancient. It cannot be a past or present contamination by the DNA of humans or other animals, which all too often is the case.

So we started looking for the right kind of monkeys among the mummified animals of ancient Egypt. Fortunately for our research, the Egyptians made mummies of pets or animals linked with gods. They worshiped many gods except during the monotheistic reign of Akhenaton, or Amenhotep IV (1353–1336 B.C.). From before pharaonic times through the Alexandrian period, an important diety was Thoth. Represented by the storklike ibis and also by a baboon, he is associated first with the sun god Ra, later with Osiris (Ra's successor), then with Horus (son of Osiris and Isis), the first pharaoh. The importance of Thoth—and therefore baboons—grew with time and the progress of Egyptian civilization. Originally Thoth was considered the inventor of speech and the tongue of creative power. He gradually became the god of writing, mathematics, and time (and thus the Egyptian calendar), as well as the moon. Finally he encompassed wisdom and civilization in general, especially their personification in the pharaoh, ruler of all Egypt.

The association of Thoth with baboons began with a cycle of myths known as "The Returning of the Eye." As with all myths, these stories are told in many versions. They are mostly imaginary but contain bits of truth and reality. The story goes that the Eye of Ra was a major source of power for the sun god. It was personified by one of his twin daughters, Tefnut, who once decided to leave her father. She traveled south to Nubia, which stretched from Aswan in Egypt to Debba in the Sudan. Nubia was inhabited by dark-skinned people. In Nubia, Tefnut changed into a lioness that terrorized humans and animals, so Ra called upon Thoth and Shu, the twin sister of Tefnut, to bring her back. They traveled through the Nubian desert disguised as monkeys. This part of the story indicates that monkeys were plentiful in Nubia because otherwise a monkey disguise would make no sense. In this disguise, Thoth found Tefnut and offered her a safe home and all the prey she wanted if she would return to Egypt. Tefnut agreed and came home to her father's welcome, accompanied by Nubian musicians and baboons. Thankful for the return of his Eye, Ra rewarded Thoth with Tefnut (who presumably had changed back to a woman). Ra also gave him the moon as his possession.

Other legends tell us more about baboons and the mummification customs so important to our research. Thoth and his wife, Nut, had a son, Osiris, whose brother Set had a different father. Thoth did not like Set and wanted his own son to be successor to Ra and ruler of Egypt. When Osiris gained the throne, he further advanced civilization, aided by Thoth. To export the new order, Osiris went to Nubia and Ethiopia, leaving Isis, his wife, as regent with Thoth. Set organized an upheaval that forced Osiris to come home, then plotted to kill him. He invited Osiris to a lavish dinner, where he displayed a large and beautiful chest in the shape of a man. As a joke, he promised to give the rule of Egypt to anyone who exactly fitted inside. One guest after another tried, and finally Osiris was convinced to try. He succeeded because Set had made the chest precisely to his measurements. But as soon as Osiris was inside, Set and his conspirators closed the lid, sealed it with molten lead, and threw the chest into the Nile. Isis mourned and searched for it along the Nile to the Mediterranean Sea. Finally, children playing on the shore told her that they had seen the chest floating out to sea. It washed up on the shores of Syria and was returned to Isis by Malacander, king of Byblos. By a miracle, Isis became pregnant by the dead Osiris, then hid with his body in the Nile Delta. Set found them, cut his brother into fourteen pieces, and scattered the pieces to all corners of Egypt.

The Egyptians believed that the dead can achieve the afterlife only when the body is preserved whole. So the faithful Isis searched and found all parts of Osiris except the penis. Aided by Thoth, she molded a new one and put all the parts together. She prepared the body for burial, laying the basis for Egyptian funeral culture and mummification. Isis then gave birth to Horus, son of Osiris, who was represented by a falcon. Thoth protected her and her son as he grew, then established Horus as the first pharaoh.

So Thoth was considered the protector of pharaonic rule, which explains why baboons are seen on pharaonic monuments, such as obelisks, as well as in temple complexes. In virtually all representations, the baboon is a male of the sacred type (*Papio hamadryas*). The baboon was seen on wall sculptures and paintings, altars, and statues. It was seen on amulets, protective charms worn by living people or buried with mummies. Sometimes the baboons are shown sitting or standing with raised paws, adoring the sun. In most cases they squat on their haunches, with forepaws on their "knees," phallus exposed. They wear a headdress adorned with full moon and crescent, and a pendant showing the eye of Ra, another symbol of

Horus. Small statues and amulets of the child Horus often show him with a baboon sitting on his shoulder. Sometimes a baboon sits on the god's disproportionately large penis, or baboons surround it. These representations seem to associate baboons and Thoth with procreation, fertility, love, or sexual fullfillment.

Whereas the sacred baboon is seen in religious art, other monkeys appear in domestic art. The ancient Egyptians were clearly familiar with various members of the Papionini tribe, mainly baboons closely related to the sacred type: the yellow baboon (*P. cynocephalus cynocephalus*), which lacks the long-haired cape of the sacred baboon, and the olive baboon (*P. c. anubis*), whose facial features are less pronounced than those of the sacred baboon. The yellow baboon and, more rarely, the olive baboon (which has greenish coloring) are common in scenes of affluent domesticity. They were apparently pets, playmates, and sometimes "watchdogs." On a wall carving from the Fifth Dynasty (2520–2360 B.C.), yellow baboons appear to be helping police by grabbing the leg of a thief in a marketplace.

More germane to our research, guenons are also seen in Egyptian art, particularly various African green monkeys. Like the yellow and olive baboons, these small monkeys were domesticated. They are shown wearing a collar or belt by which they are connected to legs of chairs or other household objects. Sometimes they are sitting under the chair of their master or mistress. African green monkeys of both sexes are seen as pets, as are female baboons, but male baboons seem reserved for religious use. Amulets showing African green monkeys often depict a monkey mother holding her child on her lap. Perhaps such amulets symbolized happy domesticity. Certainly these monkeys were popular in the decoration of domestic objects such as razors, jewel boxes, and vials for body oils and cosmetics. Most depictions show vervets or grivets, which must have been plentiful in wealthy Egyptian homes.

Most baboons and African green monkeys were probably imported from Nubia since Egyptian art often shows Nubians as guardians of these animals. A carved ebony statue from the Petrie collection, in London, represents a vervet or grivet with a woman of African appearance. An ivory statue from Mesopotamia, at the Metropolitan Museum in New York, shows an African man with one of these monkeys on his shoulder (Figure 7.1). Evidence suggests that monkeys for domestic use came up the Nile River from areas south of Nubia. However, sacred baboons came mainly from the ancient city of Punt, in what is now Eritrea. They were brought up the Red

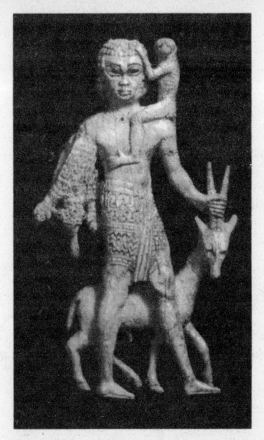

Figure 7.1   **Ancient African with monkey**. *An ivory figure from Mesopotamia, at the Metropolitan Museum in New York, represents a man with a monkey on his shoulder.* (Courtesy of the Metropolitan Museum of Art, New York.)

Sea and then through a channel to the Nile, finally reaching Memphis (Figure 7.2). A scene in the temple of Queen Hatshepsut, who ruled Egypt from 1479 to 1458 B.C., shows an expedition to Punt. Several wild-caught baboons are clearly present on the ships.

The various monkeys that came to Egypt were often mummified. This was done when a pet died, a temple animal died, or a monkey was used as a religious offering, but burial features seldom reveal their function in life. A

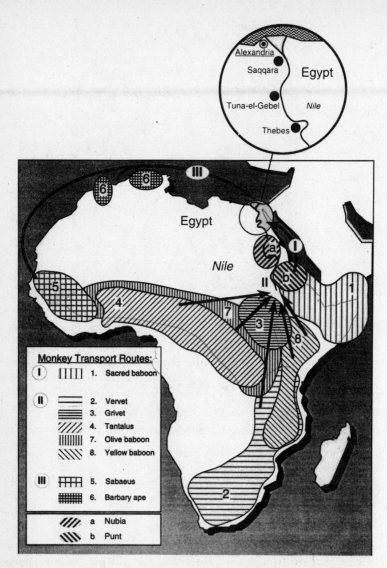

Figure 7.2 Ancient transport of monkeys and apes to Egypt. *Sabaeus monkeys and Barbary apes were imported from the west on boats that docked at Alexandria. Vervets, grivets, and olive and yellow baboons came from Nubia and farther south on the Nile River. Sacred baboons came from Punt via the Red Sea and a delta channel to the Nile, arriving at Memphis. The detail shows the main monkey mummy burial places in Egypt.* (Goudsmit and Perizonius, in prep.)

few have been found buried with humans, along with food for their journey to the afterlife. Since we have no evidence that Egyptians ate monkeys, these animals were probably not intended as food. They were more likely favorite pets. In the coffin of Queen Makare, wife of Pharaoh Pinodjem (c. 1075 B.C.), was a mummified female baboon. The pair can be seen today in the Egyptian Museum at Cairo. Museums around the world have twenty to thirty monkey skulls in their Egyptian collections, plus fourteen complete monkey mummies. They are mainly baboons but also African green monkeys.

How does one recover cell DNA, let alone viral DNA, from such specimens? The first scientific breakthrough in this research area was reported in the British journal *Nature* in 1985. Svante Pääbo, a Swedish researcher from the Wallenberg Laboratory in Uppsala, reported the molecular cloning of DNA from an ancient Egyptian human mummy. To find viral DNA—a minuscule fraction of the total DNA in blood cells—we had to replicate his work in monkeys, then extend it to the rare viral segments. We began with a human mummy, using a tiny skin scraping provided by the British Museum. The human was a male buried in a flexed position about 3300 B.C. at Gebelein, Egypt. It was chosen entirely because Svante Pääbo had been able to extract DNA from this particular mummy in 1989.

In these few cells we looked for remnants of human retroviruses that could be amplified by polymerase chain reaction (PCR). More particularly, we looked for endogenous retroviruses. How do these differ from exogenous, or infectious, viruses? Normally, retroviruses like SIV or HIV are found only in certain cell types. When endogenous, they are found in the genome of every cell of the host. This comes about when a retrovirus happens to enter a body that carries an embryo in its very earliest stage. It infects the pregnant mother in the usual way (just certain cells) but can infect *all* the embryonic cells if they are still rapidly dividing oocytes, not yet assigned their special form or function in the body. When retroviral DNA enters the genome of these undifferentiated cells, it will end up in every cell of the growing organism and, subsequently, in every cell of its progeny. The retrovirus is then endogenous, or native to that organism. The prefix *endo-* marks an insider, whereas *exo-* marks an outsider. Most endogenous viruses are relatively harmless to the host, whereas exogenous viruses (if complete) can infect the host, reproduce, and sometimes cause disease.

We looked for endogenous DNA because it is abundant, being present in every cell. This helps with PCR amplification. Abundant DNA is especially important when one works with mummies and can glean only stretches of a few hundred base pairs.

We found stretches of endogenous retrovirus that appeared to come from the mummy DNA. However, it could instead have come from the DNA of a modern human: an archaeologist, a museum curator, or a molecular biologist. Such contamination is a constant problem with mummy DNA, though we describe a partial solution later in this chapter. Because of our inconclusive results, we shifted to monkey mummies, to prove it was possible to recover ancient monkey DNA. We first used material provided by the Natural History Museum in London: a few skin cells from a small monkey, almost certainly an African green monkey and thus probably a pet. This mummy was excavated at Abydos in Egypt and dated back to the First Dynasty (2965–2815 B.C.), making it five thousand years old. As with the human mummy, DNA was recovered, but its characterization raised doubts that it was truly ancient monkey DNA. It looked more like monkey DNA than human DNA but not like the DNA of an African green monkey as shown on our genetic map of African monkey families.

More monkey material was needed and, being unavailable from a museum, was found at an animal necropolis in Egypt. Many of these animal graveyards, large and small, have been discovered by archaeologists. Extensive monkey remains are found at the three most elaborate sites: the Valley of the Queens in Thebes near Luxor, Hermopolis at Tuna-el-Gebel near Al Minya, and, finally, the Baboon Galleries of Saqqara near Giza and Cairo (Figure 7.2).

The Thebes site contains a confusion of bones and tissue of sacred baboons, yellow or olive baboons, and African green monkeys. They are all mixed together and lack any ancient or modern documentation on the frequency or distribution of types. At Tuna, remains are more organized because of the expeditions of Dieter Kessler of the Ludwig-Maximilian University and the analysis of materials by Angela von den Driesch and J. Boessneck of that same university. Most monkey mummies were olive baboons, which look very much like sacred baboons and are genetically very close. The monkey skulls at Tuna included thirteen female olive baboons, twenty-two male olive baboons, one sacred baboon, one Barbary ape, and one African green monkey. These numbers suggest strongly that olive baboons were the most frequently seen in Egypt, and that the sacred baboon was rare, even though it was favored to represent Thoth. Its very rarity could have made it seem most valuable and thus most appropriate for the god.

The monkeys at Tuna, buried in the miles-long labyrinth of underground alleys and so-called galleries, were far from healthy when they died. They included only adult or adolescent monkeys, suggesting that babies were rarely mummified. They were perhaps considered unworthy of Thoth; or perhaps the Nubians only delivered older animals. In any case, nearly all monkeys at Tuna showed signs of poor nutrition and lack of mobility. They seem to have been kept in very small cages or boxes, and their widespread tooth decay suggests they were fed sugary food considered fit for gods.

The Tuna mummies are more mixed and less well preserved than those of Saqqara, where we focused our investigation. The discovery of this site, in the Memphis necropolis, is credited to Walter Bryan Emery, who had started excavations in 1935 as an officer of the Egyptian Government Antiquities Service. After a few years he stopped because of personal and political circumstances, but he returned to northern Saqqara in 1964. In that year, by serendipity, he rediscovered catacombs containing mummies of over a million ibises. Known to early explorers and dating to 400 B.C., these Ibis Galleries were marked on maps as "Tombeaux de Momies d'Oiseaux" (Tombs of the Bird Mummies) by scientists who came to Egypt with Napoleon. However, their exact location had been lost by the end of the last century. Emery stumbled on them in an area west of the step pyramid of King Zoser (Third Dynasty: 2705–2640 B.C.).

This area is rich in the mastaba tombs of Zoser's officials, and Emery was searching for the tomb of Imhotep, architect of the step pyramid and probably also of many mastabas. The ibis catacombs suggested to Emery that he had located a pilgrimage site dedicated to Thoth. He had good reasons to expect a connection with the tomb of Imhotep since, by the time the Ibis Galleries were built, Imhotep had been deified as a god of wisdom, magic, and healing. He shared attributes with Thoth and later became identified with Thoth (and with Asklepios, Greek god of healing). In the Ptolemaic or Alexandrian period, he was even called "the image and likeness of Thoth the learned."

Emery never found the tomb of Imhotep, but in 1968 he found the Baboon Galleries. On November 23, excavations at the Saqqara necropolis reopened at the site of a small temple dedicated to Nectanebo II (360–342 B.C.). Aggressive fourth-century A.D. Christians had caused much damage, but the rubble contained many intact bronze statues, mostly representing Horus as a child. On December 7, after extensive clearing of the site, Emery found a doorway before which stood a statue of Isis nursing Horus. The doorway led to two rock-cut galleries, one above the other. At the bottom of steps to the lower gallery were two life-size limestone statues of sacred baboons. Hundreds of mummified baboons were found in the upper and lower galleries, which adjoined the Ibis Galleries. These findings told Emery that he had found a site devoted to Thoth and possibly Imhotep.

The entrance to the upper gallery is obstructed by the entrance to the lower gallery, showing that the upper was cut and filled with mummies before the lower was cut. The two galleries once contained 425 monkeys buried in niches. Emery found two intact burials, but most remains were disturbed by Christians and possibly later by robbers or treasure hunters. The animals had been mummified in a squatting position, wrapped in linen, and placed in wooden boxes. These were sealed with fine gypsum fill and placed in the niches, which were walled off with masonry or with limestone slabs. A few slabs are inscribed with the name of the monkey, its place of origin, date of burial, and sometimes the date of birth or of arrival at the temple. Some texts suggest attempts to breed baboons, since at least one baboon was said to have been born in a temple at Memphis. In general, the animals appear to have died in the temple after spending their lives there. The two limestone baboon statues found at the bottom of the steps to the lower gallery might well have decorated two limestone shrines at which ancient Egyptians perhaps offered mummified ibises and baboons or other monkeys to make their prayers convincing to Thoth.

The bones are somewhat mixed together and not yet studied in detail. They mainly represent baboons but also perhaps other monkeys. Remarkably, inscriptions on some slabs give Alexandria as the place of origin. This Mediterranean port of entry seems impossible for baboons, as well as vervets and grivets, all of which generally came up the Red Sea and the Nile. They must be Barbary apes or sabaeus monkeys, which could only have come from the western Mediterranean or through the Strait of Gibraltar from West Africa (Figure 7.2). Their importance to our research will be discussed later in this chapter.

In January 1992 the Egyptian Antiquities Organization allowed us to enter the Baboon Galleries for the first time. Led by Mohammed Attia from the University of Cairo, our team included Dutch archaeozoologist Rutger Perizonius. We found the two intact burials long gone, and the niches untouched since Emery. Still numbered by his system, they were filled with heaps of bones and skulls, as well as bits of boxes and masonry. The whole necropolis showed the devastating effect of many intruders, from Christian monks to Emery himself. According to people who worked with this archaeologist, he excavated crudely, using local workmen to clear the Baboon Galleries in just a few days.

Most of the skulls appeared to be from male baboons, but we saw smaller skulls of female baboons and other monkeys. On our visit we selected seven bones and one tooth for DNA analysis. A large right thigh bone, an upper arm bone, and the tooth belonged to one animal, a male baboon buried in a single niche. The other five bones were right thigh bones from five animals of various sizes. All samples were taken to the DNA laboratory of Attia at the National Cancer Institute in Cairo, which has been made optimally suitable for analysis of ancient DNA. Small scrapings of bone were taken from just below the neck or knob that inserts into the hip or shoulder joint. At this spot we expected the best chance of finding blood-forming tissue that might contain white cells, which in turn might contain SIV DNA. The bones and tooth were then returned to the galleries, to the niches where we found them. The scrapings were analyzed both in Egypt and in the Netherlands.

We found DNA, all right. But was it ancient DNA from a monkey or DNA from Emery and his workers? Genetic analysis of the first sample revealed it was from some kind of bird. It came from the bones of the male baboon, whose niche was near a shaft giving birds free access to the galleries. Indeed, we saw several pigeons nesting near that very niche. The DNA was possibly, but less likely, from a chicken. Participants in the Emery excavation told us that chicken was the lunch of many workers who cleared the galleries.

Besides bird DNA, the monkey bones gave us DNA that was clearly human, probably from the workmen or the archaeologists of the Emery expedition. Last but not least, many bones yielded DNA from an unknown source: not human but not monkey either. We were quickly able to rule out monkey DNA by using our genetic map for all kinds of monkeys.

We had to find the origin of these strange DNAs. If all our DNA samples were not, in fact, from the ancient monkey bones but from contemporary sources, like hatching pigeons and digging workmen, our search for ancient SIV would be nonsense.

The mystery DNA did not resemble any modern DNA, human or nonhuman, seen before by anyone. This was established by comparing it with all the stretches of DNA ever obtained by any research lab, as recorded by databases in Europe, the United States, and Japan. So, first of all, we asked ourselves if these mysterious DNA stretches were exclusively associated with ancient bones. From the National Museum of Antiquities in Leiden, the Netherlands, we obtained abdominal tissue from an intact mummified baboon from late pharaonic times. From the Smithsonian Institution in Washington, D.C., we obtained skin scrapings of red-capped mangabeys of this century (about 1917) and sooty mangabeys dating from 1896 to 1971. These ancient and modern samples revealed, again, DNA that was clearly human (pointing to contamination) plus the mystery DNA. A researcher in my laboratory, Tonja van der Kuyl, suspected that the strange DNA was also of human origin, having nothing to do with the ancient bones, teeth, or skins. She suspected it was a kind of mitochondrial DNA.

What is mitochondrial DNA? Mitochondria are energy-producing organelles that float in the cytoplasm of all human cells. Indeed, they are present in the cytoplasm of all *eukaryotes,* that is, all living things whose cells contain a nucleus. (Lower organisms like bacteria that have no nucleii are *prokaryotes.*) Mitochondria have their own "cell wall" and their own genome. This mitochondrial DNA codes for most characteristics of the organelle. It is completely independent of DNA in the nucleus, the genome of the larger organism. The nuclear DNA codes for characteristics of that organism and for a few characteristics of the organelle.

It is thought that mitochondria were originally a kind of bacterium that invaded all eukaryotes in the early stages of life on earth. They became a permanent fixture, passed down the generations of each species through the maternal lineage. (Female ova have mitochondria, but male sperm do not.) The bacterium was once a parasite, perhaps causing disease, but long ago adapted to each eukaryote species and now contributes its energy-making function.

However, over the millennia, bits of the mitochondrial DNA have migrated to the cell nucleus, where they were integrated into the nuclear DNA. So eukaryotes actually have two kinds of mitochondrial DNA: the common type that remains within the mitochondria (mtDNA) and the rare nuclear integrations. In each species the common mtDNA has coevolved with its host. In fact, its evolution is so consistent that it gives us a yardstick by which, for example, Asians, Europeans, and Americans have been traced back about 270,000 years to the "African Eve." But the nuclear integrations are stalled or frozen in time. They have not evolved with their host and therefore look much as they did when they migrated to the cell nucleus. They give us a window on the past.

Our mystery fragments appeared to be this rare type, which had dramatic consequences for our studies. Our reference map for all African primate species—like most such maps—was based on the more common and well-studied mtDNA. Such a map would be useless to identify ancient monkey DNA if both the ancient fragment and modern contaminations were primarily the nuclear integrations. We might as well be using a map of Asia to find cities and rivers of Africa. There was only one thing to do. We had to produce a new reference map based on the rare type, and so we did.

The new map showed that in human and nonhuman primates, mtDNA and its nuclear counterparts fall into two distinct clusters. All contemporary mtDNA sequences, from monkeys and other species, fall into what we may call cluster A. This also includes about half of the nuclear sequences of monkeys, but the rest fall into what we shall call cluster B. This second cluster contains, in addition, the nuclear sequences of great apes and humans.

When we matched our mystery sequences to this map, a surprising picture emerged. Although found in tissues of ancient monkeys, these sequences were identical to the nuclear integrations of humans. So people handling the samples must have shed cells that stuck to the samples, leaving this residue. Such shedding is no surprise, but why did it leave behind the rare integrations and not the more common mtDNA? The answer is that humans shed mainly skin cells. These contain very few mitochondria compared with blood cells, the cells most used in studies of mtDNA. When the shed skin cells dry up, their cytoplasm shrinks and the common mtDNA disappears, leaving only the nuclear sequences for analysis. These odd fragments remain (along with the rest of the nuclear DNA) because they are largely protected from drying by the nuclear membrane.

The mystery DNA was a blind alley in our search for ancient SIV DNA, but it raised intriguing questions. In today's search for all kinds of ancient DNA, had other researchers encountered this problem? Were there reports in the scientific literature of "ancient" DNA that was, in fact, human nuclear DNA of the mitochondrial type? Using our newly developed reference map, perhaps we could unveil the human origin of unknown sequences described by researchers working without such a map.

For example, we questioned the *Jurassic Park* scenario suggested by Woodward and coworkers. In 1994 they reported finding dinosaur DNA in fragments of large bones 80 million years old. They had found sequences they claimed were dissimilar to those of any extant species, assuming—as we had—that these sequences came from mtDNA. With this assumption in mind, Woodward thought the sequences he recovered could be nothing else than dinosaur DNA. Working with Pääbo, we investigated those sequences to see if they might instead be human nuclear integrations, that is, modern contaminations. Using human spermatozoa (which lacks mitochondria), we prepared DNA that could have only nuclear integrations of mitochondrial DNA. We used the same amplification techniques that, according to Woodward, had yielded dinosaur DNA from the large bones. We also used the putative dinosaur probes to identify the DNA. Among three thousand clones recovered from the human spermatozoa, we found three hundred positive for "dinosaur" DNA. When a family tree was drawn, this human DNA from mitochondria-free spermatozoa clustered with the DNA identified by Woodward. This result indicates that Woodward mistook human DNA for dinosaur DNA because he lacked a map for nuclear integrated mitochondrial DNA. So *Jurassic Park* is still only a story.

In any case, our problem with the mystery DNA revealed pitfalls that we could presumably avoid on our next trip to Saqqara. We had a new reference map. We also had a new and reliable technique that can confirm whether any ancient DNA whatsoever is preserved in ancient samples. Based on the fact that protein degradation parallels DNA degradation, this technique is crucial since contamination is most misleading when samples contain little or no DNA.

With these new insights we carried on with our mission: finding an SIV that caused disease in ancient times. Soon after Emery discovered the Baboon Galleries, sixteen monkey skulls were transported from there to the Petrie Museum in London. Primatologists who studied the skulls made a remarkable observation completely in line with observations at Tuna. Of the sixteen skulls, twelve were from baboons (including only four males) and two were from sabaeus monkeys or possibly tantalus monkeys. The two remaining skulls were from Barbary apes.

As noted earlier, the last four skulls are surprising since Egyptians could only have imported them from the West, through Alexandria. However, since sabaeus monkeys and Barbary apes do not overlap in their habitat, they must have been imported separately. Most important, sabaeus monkeys are the most likely species of monkey in ancient Egypt to have carried a disease-causing SIV agm, ancestor of today's SIV sm and HIV-2. But the Barbary apes are also important to our studies. Our genetic analysis revealed that these animals are very closely related to Asian macaques. In fact, it is generally assumed that all macaques in the world are descendants of Barbary apes. About six million years ago, they branched off as a separate lineage within the Papionini tribe. Once plentiful around the Mediterranean, they probably arose in North Africa and ranged into Europe as far north as England. We know this from various ancient sightings and depictions that specify a tailless monkey. The Barbary ape is the only small monkey without a tail, and the only macaque without a tail. It is also recognized by its long-haired coat, which, like its lack of tail, was an adaptation to the cold and snowy North African highlands.

Barbary apes were first reported along the North African coast by traders of the tenth century B.C. They were named for the Barbary Coast, as were the Berber people (*Barbar* in Arabic). The Barbary ape is frequently seen in ancient Greek, Etruscan, and Italian art. Aristotle distinguished this monkey from baboons and African green monkeys. Galen, the Greek physician at Rome, dissected a Barbary ape to delineate human anatomy. His model stood for hundreds of years until Vesalius finally showed that the two anatomies differ substantially.

Herodotus, the Greek historian of the Persian War, reported that the North African tribes of Gyzantes ate monkeys they captured in the North African highlands. These were most likely Barbary apes. Diodorus described the 310 B.C. expedition of Agathocles against the Carthaginians and the capture of one of the Pithecussae, or "monkey cities." The Greek for monkey is *pithekos*, and the Pithecussae were so named because monkeys were universally kept as pets. This report, confirmed by later Roman accounts, is reminiscent of West Africa, where sootys and sabaeus monkeys are used as both food and companions. Barbary apes appear to have been mainly food for the North Africans living in what are now Tunisia and Libya but mainly pets for those in Morocco and Algeria. By the nineteenth century they were extinct in the former areas and receding to isolated pockets in the latter. Today they survive in the Rif, the Moyen, and the Haut Atlas Mountains of Morocco. In Algeria they are restricted to the Chiffa and the Petite and Grande Kabylies. No Barbary apes are left in Europe, except on the Rock of Gibraltar.

At the time of the Saqqara burials (c. 400–50 B.C.), these monkeys probably ranged no farther east than the west edge of the Libyan desert, perhaps no farther than the city of Cyrene. Cursory inspection of thousands of monkey statues and pictures has found no representation of these animals. Their apparent absence from Egyptian art suggests that the two

Barbary apes of the Petrie collection—and the one from Tuna—were rare finds. The animals were apparently not used by Egyptians as pets and were offered to Thoth only as a last resort. However, they may be an important link to the disease-causing and ancestral SIV of sabaeus monkeys. They are macaques, and, as we know, Asian macaques are susceptible to AIDS-like illness at first meeting with the SIV of sooty mangabeys. Probably they are also susceptible to the related SIV agm. If Egyptians housed even a few African green monkeys with Barbary apes at their temples, they might have allowed such an encounter. They may have created a situation like the one that caused the AIDS-like epidemic among captive Asian macaques in US primate centers.

If, in ancient Egypt, a harmless SIV agm was passaged from sabaeus monkeys through Barbary apes, it might well have undergone dramatic change—exactly the kind of change we are looking for. It is not yet known whether Barbary apes now harbor SIV, or whether they would suffer AIDS-like disease if exposed to SIV sm or SIV agm. But neither is unlikely. Another possibility is that baboons in ancient Egypt were infected by SIV from African green monkeys. Passaging in baboons could have caused disease, especially since HIV-2 has been shown to cause AIDS in baboons under experimental conditions.

8

Beyond SIV and HIV:
The Cat Connection

The roots of AIDS and the AIDS virus go back before ancient Egypt and also beyond primates, as this chapter will show. But as we dig into its past, we must always remember: the virus is old and found in many species, but AIDS is new and found only in humans, with perhaps only the house cat as an odd exception. This deadly disease occurred only after harmless retroviruses of monkeys jumped, for one reason or another, to us. Instead of learning to thrive in another kind of monkey, they had to thrive in a whole new species of host. The result was three human viruses, as far as we know: HIV-0, HIV-1, and HIV-2. All cause AIDS, but each has its own history, pattern of spread, and level of lethality for the host. Of the two we know best, HIV-2 apparently had frequent passages in monkeys and needed only a few in humans to achieve optimal transmission, at small cost to the host population. In contrast, HIV-1 had rare passages in primates and needed many passages in humans to achieve optimum transmission, at much larger cost to the host population.

Clearly the history of AIDS is separate from the history of AIDS viruses. The virus just happens to cause disease in its human hosts as a side effect of optimal transmission by a given port of entry (anal or vaginal), while

causing no disease in the monkeys who gave it to humans. The development of optimal transmission and AIDS began with World War II, when
HIV-1 left its native West African habitat. It needed just a few decades to
start the Euro-American epidemic (based on anal transmission) and just a
few years more to start the epidemic in Africa (based on vaginal transmission). Both these HIV-1 epidemics have spread in Africa, Asia, Europe, and
the Americas. Meanwhile, AIDS caused by HIV-2 and HIV-0 emerged later
and remains rare because of geographic constraints, lack of opportunity,
and particular virus characteristics.

We must also remember that, like some leukemias, AIDS is simply the
result of an agent targeting a particular cell or tissue. If HIV infected less
crucial cells, as do some of its relatives, it would not be so deadly despite
the high virus load it has evolved for optimal transmission.

Keeping all this in mind, let us search back before chimpanzees (or possibly the colobus monkeys) for HIV-1 and HIV-0; and before the sooty
mangabey, the sabaeus monkey, and the vervet for HIV-2. Where did all
these monkeys get their SIVs? To find out, we must look for species that
harbor viruses like the primate viruses. However, the relatives or antece-
dents we seek may be much simpler than SIV and HIV. The primate viruses
are so complex, with all their extra genes, that one suspects those genes were
added on mainly to improve transmission, as SIV jumped along a series of
host populations or species. Those accessory genes may actually have little
to do with the potential of HIV to cause AIDS. If so, we could find a simple
nonprimate virus that has AIDS potential despite lacking those extra genes.

What nonprimate species could have given that simple virus to monkeys? The animal must have shared the monkey habitat, at least occasionally having intimate contact with monkeys. Between species, the virus
would not be transmitted sexually or perinatally but by some nonsexual
sign of affection (such as licking) or aggression (such as biting). It would be
transmitted by saliva or blood.

We will argue that certain members of the cat family are most likely,
since they shared habitat with monkeys both in Egyptian captivity and in
the East African wild. Egyptian art that depicts African green monkeys—
including sabaeus monkeys—also depicts small cats, which Egyptians are
thought to have domesticated. Monkeys may have been preferred by males
and cats by females, as suggested by the tomb painting of a man and wife
of about 1295 B.C. In this painting a monkey sits under the chair of the
man, and a cat sits under the chair of the woman. If monkeys were associ-

ated with fertility in men, as suggested earlier, perhaps cats were associated with fertility in women. In any case, monkeys and cats in the same household might sometimes become companions and groom each other. They would sometimes fight, as is proved by a tomb painting that shows a monkey jumping onto a cat under the throne of Tiy, the queen of Amenhotep III (1391–1353 B.C.). A similar fight is documented by a painting in the tomb of Neferhotep of the reign of Horemheb (1319–1307 B.C.). So more than three thousand years ago, Egyptian domestic culture gave cat viruses the chance to infect monkeys.

Did cats and monkeys also meet in the wild? As noted in Chapter 7, most monkeys imported to Egypt came from Nubia, in the south, via the Nile (olive and yellow baboons and vervets) or via the Red Sea and the Nile to Memphis (sacred baboons). Many Egyptian tomb paintings document the importation of monkeys by Nubians, or their presentation as tribute, along with other exotic animals and goods. Some show various types of monkeys and big cats together in the same scene. For example, the tomb of Rekh-mi-Re at Thebes shows Nubians offering tribute that includes a cheetah, a giraffe with an African green monkey climbing its long neck, a baboon, and a leopard. A similar scene from a Nubian temple, built by Ramses II (1290–1224 B.C.), shows an Egyptian official receiving a lion, a giraffe, two African green monkeys, and a leopard. Such representations indicate that lions, cheetahs, leopards, and monkeys shared the same habitat in East Africa and were captured alive by Nubians, or Africans living farther south, and transported to Egypt. In the wild, cats and monkeys would not show signs of affection, but they would exchange blood and saliva during conflict. Bites would be exchanged in aggression or self-defense, and sometimes a wounded monkey—infected by a cat virus—would live to spread the virus among other monkeys.

If SIV and HIV descended from cat viruses, there are two ways to look for evidence. The most cumbersome way is to study cats mummified by the Egyptians. Thousands of intact cat mummies are available in Egyptian collections all over the world, and in Egyptian burial places. Museums with large Egyptian collections generally have hundreds of cat mummies; for example, the British Museum has 244. Of all Egyptian mummified animals, cats are by far the most numerous—so numerous, in fact, that during the last century thousands and thousands were excavated, then used as fertilizer. A few of the cat mummies were swamp or jungle cats (*Felis chaus*), but most are the African wildcat (*F. silvestris libyca*), the cat assumed to be domesticated by the ancient Egyptians. Mummification of cats, like mummification of monkeys, had its peak during the Late Period (712–332 B.C.) and the subsequent Macedonian (332–305 B.C.) and Ptolemaic (305–30 B.C.) periods. Some cats were apparently killed specifically for mummification by having their necks broken when they were one to four months or nine to twelve months of age. According to Juliet Clutton-Brock of the British Museum, none of the cats in that collection lived beyond two years of age.

However, although cat mummies are more plentiful than monkey mummies, museums are not more eager to provide cat samples than monkey samples. Understandably, museums are reluctant to sacrifice any ancient material, particularly for studies that do not promise conclusive results. We are currently working with Egyptian researchers on a mummified cat family donated to our laboratory, but we also have a more promising source of evidence: the Serengeti plain in Tanzania.

Located east of Lake Victoria on the border of Tanzania with Kenya, this area became a game preserve in 1929. In 1951 a national park was established that covers the southern Serengeti and Ngorongoro areas. The Serengeti is part of the high interior plateau of East Africa. Its savannas and woodlands support the largest herds of migrating ungulates and the highest number of large predators in the world. It is a natural laboratory in which millions of wildebeests, gazelles, and zebras coexist with tens of thousands of wild dogs, hyenas, cheetahs, leopards, and lions. The primates of the Serengeti include olive baboons, colobus monkeys, and guenons; these last include patas monkeys, blue monkeys, and vervets. Baboons are infected at a very low rate with a vervet SIV. No SIV of colobus or patas monkeys has yet been found, but an SIV has been isolated from blue monkeys. Not only does it cause no disease in blue monkeys, but it causes no disease in Asian monkeys susceptible to other SIVs. Among SIVs and HIVs, the blue monkey SIV forms a separate family but, if anything, is closest to SIV agm.

Since no monkeys suffer disease from their ancestor of HIV, it seems unlikely that nonprimate species would suffer disease from an earlier and simpler ancestor. Still, such a virus could cause AIDS-like disease in one species, and not another, because of particular characteristics of that virus or its host species. So, undaunted, we look for AIDS-like disease in hooved animals and big cats. From Jembrana disease in Indonesia we know that a lentivirus of cattle (BIV) can cause a primitive form of AIDS, but does such disease occur in cattle or cats of the Serengeti? If so, is it caused by a retro-virus?

Since the nineteenth century, epidemics of deadly disease among ungu-lates have regularly occurred in the Serengeti. An 1890 epidemic affected most hooved animal species there. An epidemic from 1913 to 1921 af-fected giraffes and buffalo in particular, and epidemics of the 1930s, 1940s, and 1960s affected those two species plus the wildebeest. In all of these epidemics, the disease was characterized by an acute infection with high fevers persisting for two to three days. Then the affected animals devel-oped severe ulcers in and around the mouth, diarrhea, and discharges from eyes and nostrils. The majority of these animals subsequently wasted away and died. In the 1930s the agent was discovered to be rinderpest virus (RPV). Though not a retrovirus, it has an RNA genome. It is related to the agent of measles in humans and the canine distemper virus of dogs, foxes, ferrets, and raccoons. Other members of this virus family are deadly to por-poises, dolphins, and seals.

Recently the lions of the Serengeti park were struck by a mysterious and deadly disease, apparently a viral disease. Was the agent RPV or a re-lated RNA virus of the measles family—or could it be a retrovirus? The first death was reported in February 1994. As the year went on, about a hundred of the three thousand Serengeti lions were killed by the disease. It was not a wasting disease, as may be caused by RPV or retroviruses, but a neurological disorder manifested by seizures and paralysis of the limbs. The animals died from the progression of these neurological symptoms, which incapacitate the heart or lungs. Most often they simply cause starva-tion because the animal cannot feed itself. At first no one knew whether the infection spread from lion to lion, or to lions from prey (zebra, gazelle, or wildebeest) or a competing predator (hyenas or wild dogs). The disease looked like canine distemper, and genetic analysis of the virus linked it to a 1993 outbreak of canine distemper among big cats in California wild ani-mal parks. Lions, leopards, and tigers had succumbed in that outbreak, whose viral agent was closely related to a virus of raccoons, animals that frequently hang around zoos. However, the virus killing Serengeti lions looked less like a raccoon virus than a virus of domesticated dogs. How could this be? The most logical explanation is that domesticated dogs had given canine distemper virus to wild dogs, which gave it to lions. Wild dogs compete with lions for prey and are even sometimes eaten by lions when preferred prey, like wildebeest and gazelle, is not readily available. Apparently the canine distemper virus did not spread from lion to lion, so the deadly epidemic could be halted if lions did not meet wild dogs, or if dogs were made immune to infection.

The canine distemper virus may seem unrelated to our search, but it revealed an important clue. At the University of Rotterdam, Ab Osterhaus and colleagues inoculated the canine distemper virus of big cats into a domestic cat. Nothing happened—not the slightest sign of illness. However, further studies found that domestic cats became ill if they were already infected with feline immunodeficiency virus (FIV). As detailed in the following, this virus was discovered in a California house cat in 1987. FIV infection of cats is much less common and serious than HIV infection of people, and FIV can never be transmitted to people. But apparently it enhances the canine distemper virus load in domestic cats, just as HIV enhances the herpesvirus load in people.

If FIV made housecats more susceptible to canine distemper, perhaps a related FIV was making lions susceptible too. To look for FIV in big cats, the best way was to look for antibodies signaling past infection with such a virus. Using the FIV isolate from the California cat, Stephen O'Brien and his group at the National Cancer Institute first tested a variety of captive big cats. Among those in US and South African zoos, FIVs were found widely present in lions but only rarely present in pumas and cheetahs. No FIVs were found in lions in Asian zoos. For example, all twenty-eight lions at the Sakkarbaug Zoo in India—captured in the Gir forest in western India—were negative. However, FIV (but no disease) was found in 66 percent of the Asian lions living in American zoos. Apparently, just as monkeys in Asia never meet SIV in the wild, lions in Asia do not meet FIV in the wild—but they are susceptible when exposed. The Asiatic lions in US zoos are captive-bred descendants from five founder animals, three Asiatic lions and two African lions. Their high percentage of FIV infection must result from exposure during captivity (like Asian monkeys exposed in US primate centers) by means of sexual relations, conflict, or mother-to-child infection. The fact that the Asiatic lions suffered no ill effects from FIV of big cats shows that, unlike SIV in Asian monkeys, FIV causes no disease in new big-cat hosts.

Testing for FIV was subsequently extended to free-ranging big cats in Africa. Interestingly, FIVs were found to be widespread among cheetahs, pumas, and lions in some environments but nonexistent in other environments. FIV was found in more than three-quarters of the lions of the

Serengeti National Park of East Africa and the Kruger National Park in South Africa, but lions in southwestern Africa were negative. Similarly, Serengeti cheetahs are FIV-infected, but those of South Africa are not. The evidence indicates that the FIV infection of big cats is strongly concentrated in East Africa, particularly the Serengeti plains and woodlands.

The FIVs of house cats and big cats are clearly related, but the genetic distance between them is far greater than the distance between HIV-2 and the SIV of sooty mangabeys, or even between HIV-1 and the SIV of chimpanzees. This strongly suggests that the FIV transmission from wildcats to big cats occurred far earlier and less frequently than SIV transmission from monkeys to humans. Of course, the direction of transmission is difficult to determine for both FIV and SIV. One could argue that big cats had the virus first and gave it to wildcats—or even that monkeys gave the virus to cats, instead of the other way around. But from the genetic evidence it seems most likely that the African wildcat infected the big cats in their natural habitat. Then the big cats passed it to monkeys, who passed it to us.

Cross-species transmission might well have occurred in the Serengeti plains and woodlands where both big cats and vervets have their habitat. In this and other African preserves, the level of natural FIV infection among lions is extremely high, much higher than SIV infection among African green monkeys or sooty mangabeys. Antibodies to FIV, indicative of past infection, are found in 84 percent of lions in the Serengeti Park and 91 percent of those in the Kruger National Park. They are also found in 70 percent of lions in Ngorongoro Crater Park and 80 percent of those in Lake Manyara Park, but both populations are small. Ngorongoro Crater Park has about one hundred animals descended from fifteen founders brought in 1962 from the nearby Serengeti population to escape a disease outbreak (unrelated to FIV). Lake Manyara has an even smaller lion population, renowned because the big cats sleep in trees.

An interesting history of the big cat viruses emerges when a genealogy is constructed from FIV strains of cats in eastern and southern Africa. By analyzing one of the most conserved genes (i.e., shared by the most strains), one can see that the viruses appeared first in the Serengeti plains and woodlands, then spread to the Ngorongoro Crater, and finally to the Lake Manyara and Kruger areas. This conclusion reflects the finding by O'Brien and coworkers that the oldest group of lion FIVs contained exclusively viruses from the Serengeti, while the youngest group contained viruses from all the locales studied. So the founder virus of the East African lion population—or, for that matter, the founder virus of all African wildcats and big cats—seems to have infected first the lions of the Serengeti. The virus then spread among lions of other areas and at some point was transmitted to a monkey. Perhaps the transmitting lion did not lethally attack the monkey but only snapped or swiped at him in annoyance. Such an event would allow the monkey to survive and pass the virus to other monkeys.

Since the FIV of big cats causes no disease in its accustomed hosts, why would an FIV cause AIDS-like disease in small cats? The genetic evidence suggests that ancestral FIV evolved in two directions, affecting two distinct cat populations. Once it passed from wildcats to big cats, it evolved innocently among lions and subsequently monkeys (as SIV), spreading comfortably among these populations without causing any harm. But when wildcats were domesticated, the continuing evolution of the virus or its house cat host brought out some disease.

Apparently the house cat (*Felis catus*) is a not entirely comfortable host for FIV. However, FIV rarely causes AIDS-like disease in the domestic cat. It certainly never causes disease in humans, despite their proximity, being far too specialized for such a major cross-species jump. FIV is never such a threat to the domestic cat population as HIV is to humans. The reason for this appears to be twofold. First, FIV can spread freely among cats by its preferred route of transmission (i.e., saliva through biting) without having to increase its viral load. Second, the virus is more primitive than HIV and SIV, and lacks their genes to speed up production. Instead, it retains a primitive gene, lost by primate lentiviruses, that allows it to reproduce even in cells that are inactive. (More about this later.)

Interestingly, the house cat FIV shares all these characteristics with big-cat FIVs, which never cause disease. That the housecat FIV kills even a few of its hosts shows that a harmless virus can become harmful without changing even the slightest bit. The change can come, instead, from the evolutionary direction of the host. So far we have seen only the other pathway to disease: a virus becoming harmful by moving and adapting to a new host. Now we see that a virus can stay in the same host, but the host can change to bring out disease. In a sense, the evolution of African wildcat to house cat, as much as FIV, must be considered the cause of AIDS-like disease in cats.

FIV was found in house cats before it was even considered in big cats because it was more visible. It caused disease in animals closely and routinely observed by humans. The first case was recognized in 1987 because a woman in Petaluma, California, saw signs of something like AIDS in one of her pets. She became frustrated after taking the cat to several puzzled veterinarians. She finally brought the diseased animal to the laboratory of Niels Pedersen, a veterinary virologist at the University of California, Davis. The cat suffered from a gut infection, skin lesions, wasting, and pneumonia: all suggestive of AIDS.

Pedersen isolated a virus with similarity to the human AIDS virus. It was a retrovirus of the lentivirus family (Figure 8.1) that was genetically closer to equine infectious anemia virus (EIAV) than to the lentiviruses of ungulates or primates. In fact, the feline and equine lentiviruses are genet-

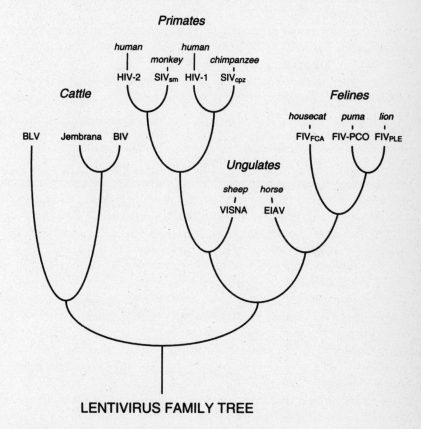

LENTIVIRUS FAMILY TREE

Figure 8.1 **Lentivirus family tree**. *Based on analysis of viral genes, the tree shows how EIAV of horses is related to FIV of house cats. It also locates the Jembrana cattle virus mentioned in Chapter 2.* (Brown et al. 1994; Chadwick et al. 1995; Omsted et al. 1992; Querat et al. 1990.)

ically equidistant from SIV and HIV. They are clustered together very
much as SIV sm is clustered with HIV-2, and SIV cpz is clustered with
HIV-0 and HIV-1 (Figure 8.2). Since the SIV/HIV clusters are thought to
imply passage between monkeys and humans, we must consider that the

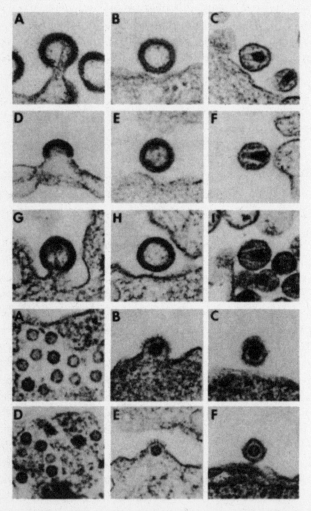

Figure 8.2 **Lentiviruses compared with other retroviruses**. *The three upper
rows show morphology of lentiviruses HIV-1 (A, B, C), HIV-2 (D, E, F), and BIV
(G, H, I). Lower rows show SFV cpz (A, B, C) and bovine foamy virus (D, E, F).
Electron micrographs by Gonda and coworkers.* (Coffin 1992; Gonda et al. 1989.)

FIV/EIAV cluster implies passage between cats and some member of the horse family. Either the cats got the virus from horses, or horses from cats. Since the FIVs of house cats and big cats have diverged farther than SIVs and HIVs have diverged, it is unlikely that house cats got their FIV from big cats, or vice versa. It is far more likely that an ancestral FIV branched in two directions, evolving with divergent populations of small cats and big cats. This ancestral FIV, carried by a wildcat or big cat, most likely came from a zebra (by biting or being bitten in defensive panic) or some ancestor of this member of the horse family.

Besides the clustering of FIV and EIAV, there is an additional reason to link the lentiviruses of cats and horses and, less so, cattle. All of these viruses are similar in lacking many genes that SIVs and HIVs gained in order to spread among primates. They also are similar in having something the primate viruses lack: a primitive gene to make the enzyme dUTPase. As we know, retroviruses can reproduce only when their host cells are activated to reproduce. Activated, or "hyperactive," host cells generate this same enzyme: dUTPase. Quiescent or resting cells do not. When SIV or HIV enters an inactive cell, it is out of luck, but the primitive lentiviruses can generate enough dUTPase to allow modest reproduction. With this capability, they can always establish infection, no matter how low their virus load or how inactive their target cells.

If an FIV-infected house cat bites another house cat, its saliva carries the virus directly into the bloodstream. Seeking white blood cells to infect, FIV ignores the CD4+ lymphocytes favored by HIV and heads instead for monocytes and macrophages. These immune cells are less crucial than CD4+ cells, which means that the infected cat suffers less illness. These cells are also less likely to be hyperactive than CD4+ cells, but the virus supplies its own dUTPase. FIV can manage with a small virus load (also good for the cat) because it can productively infect a range of cells, from hyperactive to nonactive.

FIV spreads poorly not because it cannot start infection but because it is seldom transmitted. Every bite with FIV-infected saliva will result in infection, but bites are infrequent. A house cat kept indoors is rarely bitten. Even in a multicat household, the animals normally settle disputes less aggressively. Cats usually bite other cats only when they roam and meet a territorial rival. Male cats are far more likely to get FIV-infected than females since males more readily engage in fights.

With so little chance for transmission, FIV needs the dUTPase gene to make sure no transmission is wasted. The dUTPase gene lets it multiply in any FIV-susceptible cell of monocyte lineage that it meets, active or not. Why do the primate viruses lack this apparently useful capability? A virus probably pays at least two prices for this gene. First, its virus load is reduced—but the virus should not care, since it gets more susceptible cells. Second, viral diversity is reduced. This means the host immune system can better keep up with new variants—but, again, the virus should not care if it can still spread efficiently. At some evolutionary fork in the road, the primate viruses opted for diversity: the recombination capability that, so far, overwhelms our immune system and our efforts to control AIDS.

The horse virus, so closely related to FIV, actually started the field of retrovirology. EIAV is the first retrovirus ever isolated, the first virus linked to an animal disease. In 1843, EIAV was first identified among horses in France. In 1904 its "filtrable" agent was identified, that is, an agent smaller than bacteria, not stopped by the finest filter of those days. EIAV is transmitted by bloodsucking insects that spread the virus from horse to horse. Like FIV, its target white blood cells are not the CD4+ cells but monocytes or macrophages. HIV can infect these less crucial cells but does not reproduce well in them. Aided by dUTPase, EIAV reproduces well enough to cause recurrent cycles of fever, diarrhea, and lethargy in the first year of infection. More than 90 percent of EIAV-infected horses recover and become healthy carriers of the virus for the remainder of their lives.

No one has yet tested wild horses or zebras for the presence of EIAV. However, they most likely harbor a retrovirus since, so far, retroviruses have been found in virtually every African species examined for them. African zebras live in large numbers together with buffalo and wildebeests, with whom they are prey for the lion. Geographic proximity gives viruses the opportunity to spread. The plains of the Serengeti are the habitat of buffalo, zebras, large cats, and monkeys, like the blue monkey, the vervet, and the baboon. Captive individuals of all these mammalian species have been found to share many similar viruses. Closely related viruses vary mainly in their route of transmission, especially when they have entered a new species. Success seems to hinge in part on flexibility of transmission, so a virus may spread one way within a given species (e.g., sexually) but another way (by saliva or blood) across species.

Whether or not they harbor a lentivirus, zebras surely do not get AIDS. Nor do horses get AIDS, and their lentivirus, EIAV, shares many more characteristics with FIV than with any HIV. But we can speculate that, long ago, an insect ingested blood from an EIAV-infected zebra. It next dined on a lion. Or a lion was infected while dining on a zebra, by biting or being bit-ten as the prey struggled. This EIAV strain, in becoming the founder of all FIVs, scarcely had to change its transmission route. Blood-borne in both hosts, it would enter the zebra bloodstream by an insect bite; in lions, it would enter by a zebra bite.

FIV spreads easily in lions but does not cause disease. What happened to this virus as it evolved in the house cat? Suddenly it seems to be causing sporadic but dreadful disease. Has it truly just started, or have we only just noticed? Can it truly cause AIDS-like disease, by itself, or does disease oc-cur only under certain well-controlled and forced circumstances?

FIV is present in about 1 percent of domestic cats in Europe, the United States, and Australia. In some isolated pockets, notably Japan, its incidence is slightly higher. In a given area the incidence never rises, so it never reaches epidemic proportions. In general, incidence is low and promises to remain low. It is surprising that house cat FIV is relatively high in Asia, since Asian big cats have no FIV (and Asian monkeys have no SIV). But this can be seen as more evidence that the FIV of house cats long ago diverged from the FIV of big cats. It also confirms that house cats are a relatively new and unaccustomed host for FIV.

There is clear evidence that FIV, on its own, can cause AIDS-like dis-ease. Plasma containing the virus was taken from house cats during the ini-tial acute stage of FIV infection. This was injected into cats a few weeks old, resulting in FIV infection with a dramatic course never seen before. It looked just like AIDS: the animals had diarrhea, wasting, decreased CD4+ cell numbers, and virus in all parts of the body. More than half died within two months of infection. This proves beyond a doubt that FIV has the po-tential to cause an immunodeficiency under optimal conditions. However, in real life it seldom gets such conditions. If it gets into the bloodstream, it infects each and every new host, but it rarely gets there. And since passage of any kind is rare, passage during the acute phase of infection (which lasts only one or two weeks) has to be considered the rarest of all rare events. The transmission of FIV among house cats is infrequent, and disease is even more infrequent. If many cats were suffering so-called AIDS in peo-ple's homes, we would know about it from veterinarians. Given the fear of human AIDS, we would read about a cat epidemic in the newspapers, even though FIV or its infection could never harm humans. In centuries of living close to humans, a cat virus would have invaded us long ago if we were suitable hosts.

The important point is that although FIV alone can cause AIDS-like disease and premature death in cats, it rarely does so, except under experimental conditions. When cats appear to suffer such an outcome in natural surroundings, it must usually be ascribed to other cat retroviruses that infected the animal simultaneously. FIV alone can eventually damage the feline immune system but not so efficiently as HIV can damage ours. Cats are much more threatened by another virus that can cause AIDS-like disease as well as leukemias: feline leukemia virus (FeLV).

FeLV was discovered in Scotland in 1964 by Bill Jarrett as the cause of feline leukemia. It is a very rudimentary retrovirus that lacks even the extra genes of simple lentiviruses like FIV, including the dUTPase gene. The FeLV genome has only three genes: one to encode for enzymes that splice it into host DNA, two to package the RNA molecules and enzymes in a particle. But they get the job done. FeLV is a versatile virus that retained the capacity to cause immunodeficiency as it evolved to cause cancers. Certain strains of FeLV cause AIDS-like disease in all species of animals experimentally infected. Of course, organisms often grow more readily under experimental conditions than in life. In vitro, especially on cell lines, they can be made to grow where they would never grow in vivo. Feline leukemia virus can infect human cell lines but, as noted, has never infected humans in the real world.

Lions and cheetahs are never infected by FeLV. Either this virus has never been introduced to these populations or it is unable to infect them. This last alternative is not far-fetched since lions and cheetahs lack endogenous FeLV. This shows that the virus never could infect them, even in ancient times. In contrast, endogenous FeLV is found in all the cells, including blood cells, of the domestic cat and its wild relatives and ancestors, the jungle cat and wildcat.

If one speculates that AIDS-like disease in house cats is the result of FeLV infection, alone or in combination with FIV, one would expect never to see the disease in lions and cheetahs, since they get FIV but never FeLV. And that is exactly the case: the disease is restricted to house cats and never observed in big cats.

Feline leukemia virus infects house cats in their early years: more than 50 percent are infected before the age of five. In contrast, FIV infects them later: more than 50 percent are infected after the age of five. In the average multiple-cat household, about one-third are FeLV-infected, though not all will show disease. In a similar household, a much smaller fraction is infected with FIV. This confirms that FeLV spreads better, being transmitted by licking and grooming, whereas FIV requires biting.

FIV alone causes negligible mortality, but FeLV alone has a dramatic effect on the life span of an infected cat. A study of multiple-cat households found that over a period of 3.5 years, mortality was 83 percent among cats infected with FeLV but only 16 percent among those not infected with the virus. The deaths were caused mainly by FeLV-induced immunodeficiency and the clinical manifestations of feline AIDS. A minority of the infected cats died of other FeLV-related diseases like anemia and lymphoid tumors.

Feline AIDS due to FeLV infection is indistinguishable from feline AIDS due to the very rare cases of FIV infection. FeLV replicates in cells of the immune system and causes functional as well as numerical abnormalities of T cells. These abnormalities occur before signs of disease are clinically apparent. In FeLV-infected cats, FIV behaves very much as an opportunistic infection. FeLV has been shown to enhance the infectivity of FIV by making the host apparently more susceptible to its invasion. FeLV-infected cats are much more likely to be infected by FIV, when exposed, than cats not infected with FeLV.

When cats are infected with FeLV and then FIV, their immunodeficiency and disease are more severe—and death occurs sooner—than in animals infected with FeLV alone. But the reverse is not true. When healthy FIV-infected cats become infected with FeLV, the disease course runs pretty much as in cats without FIV. These data strongly indicate that FeLV causes AIDS on its own and poses a life threat to cats in their natural surroundings; but FIV alone is little threat (despite its established AIDS potential), and in most natural cases can only deepen the immune suppression caused by FeLV. Nevertheless, while FIV is relatively harmless alone, it must be considered the worst of all opportunistic infections affecting cats immunosuppressed by FeLV. The opportunistic damage of FIV most likely depends on FeLV activation of FIV-susceptible cells. FIV can then increase its usually modest production; it can aggravate FeLV-associated immunodeficiency and its clinical manifestations.

The "cooperation" of these two viruses clearly benefits FIV, but what about FeLV? Like FIV, its survival depends on spread, yet by enhancing FIV production, the leukemia virus hastens the death of the host. The answer may lie in the fact that the two viruses can infect the same feline white blood cells. Dual infection of these cells has occurred in vitro, resulting in viable recombinants of FIV and FeLV. So perhaps the advantage for FeLV lies in diversity. If FeLV increases the chance of FIV infection, it also increases the chance of dual infection, viral sex, and recombination. FeLV seems highly successful, but the availability of FIV provides options if needed. If new circumstances threaten, FeLV genes might survive in a recombinant having FIV's ability to manufacture dUTPase or spread by biting. A recombinant might appear with brand-new characteristics: the ability to enter a new target cell or even a new host.

The lentivirus of cattle (BIV) or horses (EIAV) apparently infected wildcats or big cats (FIV), then lions infected monkeys (SIV) and monkeys infected humans (HIV), while wildcats evolved into house cats (FIV). Though all related (Figure 8.1), these retroviruses have no AIDS potential—or even much disease potential—except in house cats, Asian monkeys, and humans. However, in cats we see not one but two retroviruses that can cause AIDS-like disease: FIV and FeLV. Despite its relationship to HIV, FIV rarely does harm without special circumstances, because it generally spreads enough for survival. The rudimentary FeLV is more aggressive. It frequently causes feline AIDS and also facilitates the spread of FIV. Its cooperation with FIV hastens deterioration of the host but may give FeLV the benefit of diversity.

We are lucky that HIV has not teamed up with such a helpful virus. Or has it? If FeLV helps FIV in house cats, need we fear such an ominous partnership between the more complex retroviruses of monkeys and humans?

9

The Mystery Suitor:
HIV's Next Move

It is not enough to know HIV and its past incarnations. We must use what we know to anticipate—and perhaps manipulate—the future of this virus. Major leaps in retrovirus evolution happen because distinct retroviruses engage in sex and recombination. Sexual reproduction demands a partner, but not every partner suits SIV or HIV. It must be a retrovirus with sufficient stretches of genetic similarity to enable the production of offspring. It must share the same taste, infecting the same target cell of the same species of host. Last but not least, it must be available—for how can the partners possibly mate if they never meet?

Already we see that sex and recombination have happened many times between AIDS viruses to yield new viruses, the most notorious being HIV-1E. This is the offspring of HIV-1A and another HIV-1 parent that, if still extant, is so rare that nobody has found it. HIV-1E is so viable that it has spread rapidly in Asia and become the predominant cause of AIDS on that enormously populated continent. But its parents were close relatives, so their mating did not cause a major evolutionary leap. If a retrovirus needs new genes to survive, it must find a mate outside its immediate family.

A likely suitor for SIV or HIV must be a retrovirus that circulates in the same primate populations, but cocirculation is not enough. Two viruses must not only share locale and host but meet in the same hyperactive target cell at about the same time. They must establish a dual infection in that cell, which can happen two ways. Either the partners enter the cell simultaneously, which is called *coinfection,* or one partner enters and is later joined by a second, which is called *superinfection.* Only the first way is possible for viruses that have the same target cell and enter by the same receptor molecule. This is because viruses that use the same receptor compete for entry. In general, they can both enter if they arrive at the same instant. But if one beats the other, it may enter and remove the receptor, like a man who climbs a rope ladder and then takes it away with him. The first arrival thus prevents superinfection by a latecomer that needs the same receptor. HIV uses this strategy, which minimizes sex within the family. As soon as one HIV infects a T cell, the surface CD4 molecules are dramatically reduced, making the cell difficult or impossible to infect by a second HIV strain.

This phenomenon, called *superinfection interference,* is an almost universal reproductive strategy among mammals. Of the millions of spermatozoa that compete to fertilize an egg, a single one succeeds and immediately makes it impossible for other sperm to enter the egg. With retroviruses, it seems that when a virus begins adaptation to a given set of conditions, the door is wide open for sex. Coinfection or superinfection can easily take place. But as soon as that virus nears optimal adaptation for spread in the host at hand, the opportunities for sex become limited to coinfecting partners. These partners need donor hosts who deliver them simultaneously to the new hosts, which requires (among other things) the same route of infection. The coinfection system seems to represent fine-tuning at the end stage of the adaptation process. It is the finishing touch for a retrovirus that has, at least for the moment, won the viral wars and mastered its conditions of spread. Superinfection interference appears to have evolved to slow down the pace of recombination when the future looks bright for the virus in its niche.

But until that bright future is achieved, or when it is someday threatened by a changed environment, superinfection interference is counterproductive. The retrovirus will become extinct if unable to mate with a partner that can contribute the survival gene. Apparently, superinfection interference cannot be repealed, so the threatened virus needs a new kind of partner: one that enters the same target cell but uses an entirely different receptor molecule. Using distinct receptors, two viruses can enter a cell without superinfection interference. They need not be simultaneously transmitted, by the same route, in order to mate. One virus can infect a cell and simply wait for its potential partner to arrive.

So our real search is for a retrovirus that infects the same human lymphocytes as HIV—the T cells that carry the CD4 molecule—but uses another molecule to enter those cells. Is there a known retrovirus that fits this description? Even more frightening, has this mystery retrovirus already been seen to superinfect monkeys or humans with SIV or HIV?

So far we know of seven candidates: seven groups of retroviruses that infect humans and other animals. (Remember that plant viruses cannot infect animals.) Four are relatively simple, and three are more complex. Of the simple four, only two can infect any human cells: a group of cat viruses including FeLV, and a group of monkey viruses, for example, MPMV, BaEV, and GALV (discussed in Chapter 10). But none of these has shown human disease potential and, more important, none infects the target cells of SIV or HIV. The same is true of one of the three complex groups, the spumaviruses (from *spume*, "spray," because they cause vacuolization, or foaming, of cells in culture). However, the other two complex groups could supply a suitor. They are the primate lentiviruses (SIV and HIV) and the primate tumor viruses. A lentivirus suitor would not produce a big evolutionary leap. That leaves the tumor viruses, more specifically known as T-cell lymphoma/leukemia viruses. In humans they are called HTLV; in simians, STLV.

These retroviruses were discovered at the end of the 1970s, a decade when researchers worldwide were looking for a cancer virus of humans. By then, retroviruses had been identified as the cause of cancers in chicken, turkeys, mice, rats, and cats—but not in humans. On top of the research list were tumors of white blood cells: leukemias and lymphomas. United States and European researchers concentrated their attention on T-cell lymphomas of the skin, specifically mycosis fungoides and Sézary syndrome. Japanese investigators were most interested in a form of blood cancer, adult T-cell leukemia, which has a mysteriously high incidence on the southern Japanese island of Kyushu.

In the Netherlands a small research group in the Pathology Laboratory of Leiden University Medical Center focused on retroviruses as a putative cause of human cancers. The researchers mastered a new technology that was pivotal to their success. It allowed them to detect reverse transcriptase activity not only within infected cells but in cell-free virions, that is, retrovirus particles circulating in extracellular space. In 1979, one year before US and Japanese groups reported similar and more refined observations, Elizabeth van der Loo and Chris Meyer reported an intriguing series of experiments in an obscure journal (*Virchows Arch. B. Cell Pathol.*, 31, 193–203). They had studied seven patients with mycosis fungoides and two with Sézary syndrome as well as eight controls: patients with unrelated skin diseases.

Particles that looked like retrovirus particles were found by electron microscopy in skin biopsies of all nine patients with the T-cell cutaneous lymphoma but in none of the controls (Figure 9.1a,b). The lymph nodes of four tumor patients were examined and found to contain the same virions, an indication of generalized infection. Van der Loo went on to show that these virions had a dense round core, typical of C-type retroviruses. The virions were invariably found in Langerhans' cells. These immune cells of the skin also occur in vaginal tissue, where they are attacked by HIV, as mentioned earlier.

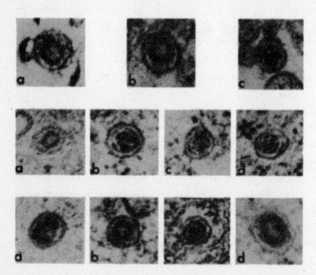

Figure 9.1a *Electron micrographs of the retrovirus particles observed by van der Loo and Meyer in 1979.* (van der Loo et al. 1979)

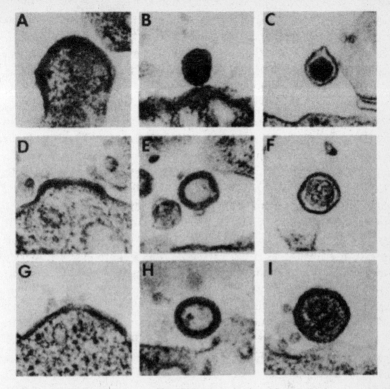

Figure 9.1b   *Electron micrographs of HTLV and related bovine leukemia virus, by Gonda and coworkers.* (Coffin 1992; Gonda et al. 1989)

So van der Loo had shown a virus to be present, but was it a retrovirus, as she suspected? Was it incidental to the lymphoma or directly related to its etiology? Knowing she needed more proof, she extracted virions from the skin lesion of one tumor patient and showed them to have a density of 1.16 g/cm^3 when intact. This density corresponds exactly to C-type retroviruses, and under electron microscopy the virions were indistinguishable from those seen in the Langerhans' cells of the patient. As final proof, van der Loo tested for the presence of reverse transcriptase. She detected its activity only in the tumor patients and only in the virions of 1.16 g/cm^3 density, not in material of any other density. No activity was found in material from the lesions of control patients. Thus van der Loo showed particles with all the characteristics of C-type retroviruses to be present in immune cells of the skin and interdigitating cells of the lymph nodes. (These are cells of the same family that interlace with others by extending protrusions around them.) On top of that, she showed that purified particles had reverse transcriptase sequestered at their core.

Based on all these results, van der Loo cautiously concluded that if these lymphoma patients had particles like C-type retroviruses in cells with a preference for T-cell regions, those particles might be related to the cause or development of the lymphoma. Like any good scientist, van der Loo was cautious to avoid reasoning *post hoc propter hoc*: if X occurs after Y, it must be *caused* by Y. (Or, more generally, if two things occur together, one must influence the other in some way.) But although her conclusion lacked formal proof, it is now widely accepted.

In 1980 Bernard Poiesz and Bob Gallo propagated the virus-producing T cells of patients with T-cell cutaneous lymphomas. They then isolated the retrovirus that would be known as HTLV. In 1981 and 1982, respectively, Hinuma and Yoshida isolated the same retrovirus from T-cell lines derived from patients with adult T-cell leukemia. All strains were shown to belong to the same family of human C-type retroviruses. One of Yoshida's cell lines, which is persistently infected with HTLV, soon became the cell line of choice to determine biological differences among HIV-1 viruses. Named MT-2, it was found to be readily superinfected by aggressive HIV-1 strains isolated from rapidly deteriorating patients, but not by HIV-1 strains from healthy and recently infected individuals. Already, in those early days, we had our first ominous clue that an HTLV-infected individual might select for (i.e., favor infection by) more aggressive HIV strains.

Later in 1982 the Gallo group found a second member of the HTLV family in a patient with hairy cell leukemia, another rare cancer of white blood cells. This virus was immediately called HTLV-II, and the previously discovered virus became HTLV-I. These two retroviruses are members of the same virus family, related much like HIV-1 and HIV-2. They have simian counterparts, STLV-I and STLV-II. Interestingly, the viruses of Old World monkeys and apes (STLV-I) cluster with HTLV-I, whereas those of New World animals (STLV-II) cluster with HTLV-II.

The tumor viruses are grouped with oncoviruses, or cancer viruses. However, disease is associated very rarely with HTLV-I and even more rarely with HTLV-II. Infection by HTLV-I develops into adult T-cell leukemia or other lymphomas in perhaps one out of a thousand infected individuals.

Even then, disease occurs many decades after infection is acquired. The main route of transmission is ingestion of breast milk, so infections tend to remain limited to families with HTLV-I-positive females of childbearing age. Infection can readily be prevented by heating or freeze-thawing the milk of positive mothers before giving it to their children. In rare cases the virus has been acquired by bottle-fed babies, indicating that it can be transmitted by the intrauterine or vaginal route, albeit seldom. Clusters of HTLV-I infections appear to occur when the sons of positive mothers are infected by breast milk and, as adults, pass the virus to spouses during vaginal intercourse. The spouses then infect their offspring by breastfeeding, and so on.

Though males can sexually transmit HTLV to females, the opposite is rare. This is because only HTLV-I-infected cells are contagious, not cell-free virus particles; and the infected cells are much more plentiful in semen and blood than in vaginal fluids. The rarity of female-to-male transmission hampers the spread of HTLV-I and appears to explain the absence of epidemic adult T-cell leukemia. Moreover, the virus does not spread by anal transmission, so it cannot follow the path taken by HIV-1B in starting the AIDS epidemic in Europe and the United States. At first glance this is surprising because HIV and HTLV-I can infect the same CD4+ cells in vitro. However, in vivo, HTLV-I is apparently unable to infect the Langerhans' cells of the anal or lower-intestinal mucosal wall. HIV attacks such cells with cell-free particles, which in HTLV-1 are relatively few and harmless.

At one time in the early 1980s, HTLV-I was seen as a possible cause of AIDS. When the Pasteur group announced the finding of HIV in *Science* (Barré-Sinoussi, 1983), the very same issue carried three articles by Essex et al. from Harvard and Gallo et al. from the National Cancer Institute linking AIDS with HTLV-I. The Essex group had found antibodies to the virus in nineteen of seventy-five AIDS patients (39 percent), but the Gallo group, testing for HTLV-I DNA in peripheral blood lymphocytes, had found it in only two of thirty-three AIDS patients (6 percent). Gallo's results suggest that the test used by Essex scored many AIDS patients false-positive for HTLV-I. The results of both Gallo and Essex suggest that HTLV-I could not be the cause of AIDS since it was not found in all, or even the majority, of the AIDS patients studied.

Most important to this discussion, their results suggest that HIV and a tumor virus had already established double infections (if only rarely) at the very onset of the first major AIDS epidemic. Subsequent work has found 5 to 10 percent of AIDS patients to be infected by HTLV-I or HTLV-II. They are mainly gay men, which was initially puzzling since the virus does not transmit by the anogenital route. In 1987 some clues emerged from a study we did among homosexual men in Amsterdam. Only 3 of 697 healthy homosexual men (0.4 percent) were HTLV-I-positive in 1984, and two more became positive over the next two years: not much of an epidemic, one would say. Interestingly, one of the first three individuals was a Brazilian, and one of the next two acquired the virus after relations with a Brazilian during a holiday in Brazil. These data indicate that, in the risk group we were studying, HTLV-I was imported from South America. In addition, our data suggest that orogenital, not anogenital, relations had caused the HTLV-I infection. This observation is consistent with the main route of HTLV-I infection: breastmilk ingestion. Apparently fluids containing HTLV-I-infected cells must contact cells in the mouth and throat in order to infect a new host.

So the bad news is that HTLV-I and HIV both infect our CD4+ cells. And HTLV uses another entry molecule, not yet known. The good news is that they rarely infect the same individual and, when they do, they infect CD4+ cells in different parts of the body. This is because HIV primarily enters the body through cells of the anal or vaginal wall, whereas HTLV-I enters by cells of the mouth and throat. This puts them at opposite ends of the twenty-six-foot alimentary tract, making sex and recombination difficult. In theory, double infection can occur. After entry, both viruses infect CD4+ cells that circulate around the body, so, for example, HIV could enter anally and infect a cell that makes its way to the throat, where HTLV is available. But in practice this meeting is unlikely, especially since CD4+ cells have a limited life span.

If gay men are not likely to bring these two viruses together, will some other host be a better matchmaker? We have begun to test for HTLV-I in the Netherlands and have found the virus in people from Suriname and Brazil in South America, from the Caribbean, and from northwestern Africa. This suggests that HTLV circulates in their countries of origin, as indeed it does. Whether Netherlanders not from those origins might also carry HTLV has not yet been determined.

HTLV-I has a patchy and apparently random distribution compared with HIV-1. In Japan it is endemic among the Ainu people on the island of

Hokkaido in the north, among the Ryukyuan of Okinawa in the extreme south, and on the island of Kyushu. It causes disease only in the last region, where it causes adult T-cell leukemia. This indicates a special strain of HTLV, as explained toward the end of this chapter.

Except perhaps in southern India, HTLV-I has no significant presence in the rest of Asia, not even in the Japanese neighbors of Korea and China. Looking farther afield, David Asher and D. Carleton Gajdusek of the National Institutes of Health, together with my own group, tested one thousand individuals from fourteen populations of the southwestern Pacific. This oceanic survey found HTLV-I to be endemic among Melanesians living in the coastal lowlands of Papua New Guinea, on the northern New Guinea islands and on the Torres and Banks Islands, as well as among Polynesians living on the Solomon Islands. When publishing these findings, we presented evidence that these Pacific strains may be different from the strains in Kyushu, the Americas, and the Caribbean. This has turned out to be the case.

Other researchers have shown HTLV-I to be present along the western coast of Africa in such countries as Morocco, Mauritania, Senegal, Guinea-Bissau, Liberia, Ivory Coast, Ghana, and as far south as Gabon and Zaire. But its presence among inhabitants of East Africa appears to be extremely low. In the Americas, HTLV-I is found among African-Americans in the southern states of the United States. It is found in blacks of the Caribbean and in blacks and indigenous peoples of the northern countries of South America, such as Peru, Brazil, and Suriname. It is also found among Alaskan Eskimos and British Columbian Indians.

This erratic distribution can be explained, but first we must take a detour. We must discuss HTLV-II (though it is less urgent to our search) and the simian tumor viruses, and why all this distribution is important. HTLV-II is endemic in Mongolia in Asia, among Alaskan Eskimos, and among other Amerindian populations living farther south in the Americas. In Africa, HTLV-II is present in remote forest areas of Zaire, Cameroon, and Gabon, primarily among the forest people but also in large towns of Ghana and Cameroon. As noted later, we suspect an ancient transfer of the virus to the remote areas, and a more recent transfer to the city areas.

STLV-II has not yet been found in Africa but is seen in New World monkeys. As noted previously, STLV-II viruses cluster together with HTLV-II viruses and apart from viruses of the HTLV-I group and STLV-I.

STLV-I viruses are widespread around the globe, except among New World monkeys. Not all species of Old World monkeys carry STLV-I, but many more than carry SIV. Like SIV, it is usually harmless, but its prevalence among STLV-I-susceptible species is higher than the prevalence of SIV among SIV-susceptible species. And unlike SIV, it infects not only African monkeys in the wild but also Asian monkeys in the wild. Since Asian monkeys are accustomed to it, STLV-I does not make them sick. Asian monkeys infected with this virus include macaques from Japan and its islands (*Macaca fuscata*), except the island of Hokkaido. They also include macaques from Indonesia (*Macaca fascicularis*) and India (*Macaca mulatta*). STLV-I has not been found in Asian colobus monkeys or gibbons.

In Africa, STLV-I parallels SIV in infecting all four subspecies of African green monkey (sabaeus monkeys, grivets, vervets, and tantalus monkeys), mandrills, and sooty mangabeys (but no other mangabeys). In addition, STLV-I is highly prevalent in many more guenons: the blue monkey (*Cercopithecus mitis*), crowned guenon (*Cercopithecus mona pogonias*), and patas monkey (*Cercopithecus patas*), as well as olive, yellow, and sacred baboons. This virus is also found in chimpanzees and gorillas. Interestingly, although it appears to infect baboons and African green monkeys, it does not infect the other species we saw in the Egyptian Baboon Galleries: the Barbary ape. When Gerhard Hunsmann tested primates in 1983, as did Poiesz in 1994, not a single STLV-I-positive Barbary ape was found among one hundred tested.

In conclusion, STLV-I appears to be highly endemic among Asian macaques, four groups of African guenons (African green monkeys, patas monkeys, blue monkeys, and crowned guenons), baboons, and mandrills. Infected chimpanzees and gorillas appear to be quite a rare find in the wild. So one might say that STLV-I pervades two large families of Old World monkeys: the guenons and the Papionini tribe. SIV is prevalent in exactly the same two families, but in fewer species, and not in Asia.

As shown in Figure 9.2, pockets exist in Africa—particularly central and western Africa—where SIV cocirculates with STLV-I, and HIV cocirculates with HTLV-I. In addition, HTLV-II circulates with HIV-0 in Cameroon and Gabon. Both HTLV-I and HTLV-II circulate with HIV-1 in central Africa, and with HIV-2 in West Africa. Is this a problem? Does it matter that these tumor viruses have migrated and come to circulate with SIVs and HIVs? After all, cocirculation does not always lead to dual infec-

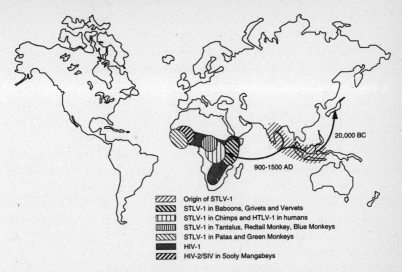

Figure 9.2   Travels and distribution of simian T-cell leukemia virus type I.
Imported from Asia, STLV-I appears to have moved east to west across Africa, in-
fecting various monkey hosts including chimpanzees, from which it finally
crossed to humans as HTLV-I. (Chen et al. 1995; Fultz et al. 1990; Hunsmann
et al. 1993; Koralnik et al. 1994; Saksena et al. 1994.)

tion and disease or recombinants. Have these viruses ever actually met SIV
or HIV in the same target cells in the same part of the same host, human or
simian, with any ill effects?

While anal sex rarely if ever transmits HTLV-I or HTLV-II, gay men
sometimes acquire HTLV-II when taking IV drugs. Among drug users in
general, gay or straight, dual infections of HTLV-II with HIV are not uncommon. This is because all HIVs and both HTLVs are efficiently transmitted by blood cells. When injected directly into the bloodstream, they
can bypass anal or vaginal entry, for which HTLV is ill equipped.

Another ominous note is that given HTLV-I's endemicity—in the populations of Haiti in the Caribbean, for example, and Guinea-Bissau in West
Africa—double infections by HIV and HTLV-I are much more common
than expected on the basis of the frequency of either virus alone. This adds
to evidence, mentioned earlier, that infection by one of these viruses facilitates infection by the other. The same appears to be true for their simian

counterparts. Double infection by STLV-I and SIV is not uncommon among mandrills in a breeding colony of the International Medical Research Center in Franceville, Gabon, or among sooty mangabeys at the Yerkes Primate Research Center of Emory University in Atlanta, Georgia.

In virtually all cases so far, such double infections have been harmless, causing no adult T-cell leukemia in humans or monkeys. Double infection rarely if ever occurs in the Papionini tribe. However, a totally different picture has emerged from investigation of African green monkeys.

In Senegal, STLV-I and SIV infections have been extensively studied in two discrete areas that are 600 kilometers apart. One is the forested savanna region of Kedougou in southeastern Senegal near the Guinean border. The other is the savanna region of Sine-Saloum in central Senegal near the border with the Gambia. The Kedougou studies occurred during a yellow fever control campaign in 1981 and 1982, and included 120 wild-caught monkeys. The Sine-Saloum studies took place more recently, in 1989 and 1991, and included 51 monkeys. It is known that in these two separate regions of Senegal, more than one of every three patas monkeys is infected with STLV-I. Of course, patas monkeys are rarely, if ever, infected with SIV. But of sabaeus monkeys in these two areas, STLV-I infects more than 35 percent—as does SIV—and about 22 percent are infected with both viruses. A monkey already infected with the tumor virus has a more than 50 percent chance of acquiring an SIV infection as well.

Moreover, whereas HTLV-I appears to spread among humans mainly by breast milk or blood, the STLV-I of green monkeys appears to have learned how to spread sexually. This also appears to be true for STLV-I among other guenons and the Papionini tribe. Among mandrills of the breeding colony in Gabon, only adult males were documented to be STLV-I positive, and such males acquired SIV either simultaneously with STLV-I infection or years afterward. This study does not rule out infection through aggression during territorial fights, as occurs with FIV. However, among all guenons studied in the wild, adult females are as frequently positive as males. This argues against infection by fighting (in which females are rarely involved) and underlines sexual contact as the main route of transmission among sabaeus monkeys and probably other types of African green monkey.

By itself, STLV-I does not appear to cause disease in African green monkeys, nor does SIV. Two cases, however, indicate that the combination of these two viruses can be quite deadly. Hayami from Kyoto University has described the development of lymphoma caused by an aggressive STLV-I in an SIV-infected African green monkey. This suggested that a double infection of these two viruses can spur STLV-I to attack the host. Mickey Murphey-Corb described an even more stunning case from the Tulane Regional Primate Research Center at Covington, Louisiana. A female African green monkey, born ten years earlier in the wild, suddenly developed a wasting disease reminiscent of that seen in Asian macaques experimentally infected with SIV. Besides opportunistic infections, this monkey showed dramatic enlargement of lymph nodes all over her body. This sudden proliferation of lymphoid cells was caused by STLV-I, which had been integrated into cells hyperactivated by SIV. It remains to be seen whether these cases are flukes or ominous warnings of new types of retroviral disease.

At one time, STLV and HTLV did not seem able to infect the same cells in the same region of the body as SIV and HIV. And as long as the tumor viruses stayed in Asia and the Pacific, and HIV and SIV stayed Africa, what could go wrong? But apparently a lot has changed over the last few hundred years. STLV moved from Asia to Africa, and HTLV moved from Asia to both Africa and the Americas. At the same time, SIV and HIV moved around in Africa. HIV, if not SIV, spread to the Americas and Asia. These changes in distribution brought the two families together among both the monkeys and the humans of Africa. Double infection leading to recombinants could occur in either case but is currently more threatening in monkeys.

So far, HTLV still appears to favor oral transmission. Our results from gay men of Amsterdam indicate that HIV and HTLV are still not infecting the very same host cells. In monkeys, however, we see that STLV has acquired the same mode of transmission as SIV. Both are spread sexually among adult monkeys, so both can infect cells of the same body regions.

This sets the stage for new viruses to emerge from the cohabitation of STLV and SIV. The first steps have been taken: the viruses cocirculate in the same habitat and geographic areas and infect the same hosts by the same route. Double infection appears to be more harmful than a single retrovirus infection. In one instance, STLV added to SIV has already brought out a clinically apparent immunodeficiency; in another, it has brought out an aggresssive lymphoma. STLV/SIV recombinants have not yet been seen, but they may have occurred and simply not survived. More truly viable recombinants may only await formation of those rare offspring with the necessary advantages. And from the history of SIV and HIV, we know that simian viruses can find their way into the human population.

Migrations of Tumor Viruses

Distribution and cocirculation definitely matter, but how did STLV-I get into Africa in the first place? How did HTLV-I get into isolated populations like the Ainu and the people of Okinawa and Kyushu? Why do only Kyushu-type strains cause adult T-cell leukemia? HTLV-I strains in Melanesia and Polynesia appear to belong to a group of relatively innocent viruses. Strains from Africa, the Caribbean, and the Americas seem related to the Kyushu strains. Apparently the migration history of the tumor viruses is at least as complicated as that of SIV and HIV, and a great deal older. Unlike SIV and HIV, the STLVs and HTLVs seem to have sailed separate courses for a very long time. Even among the human tumor viruses, we see completely separate lineages and histories.

The family tree of these retroviruses appears to have many large and small branches. The oldest member of the family appears to be a bovine leukemia virus, which gave rise to two main branches. On one branch we see STLV-II and HTLV-II, which infect New World monkeys and New World humans, including Amerindians. The latter was only recently noted in the Old World (in Africa), long after its endemicity had been demonstrated in the New World. HTLV-II strains are found in both North and South America, in West and equatorial Africa, and practically nowhere else. Currently, HTLV-II spreads particularly among IV drug users in the United States, who are frequently infected by both HTLV-II and HIV. But these infections have little relevance to our story because HTLV-II mainly infects CD8-positive (CD8+) cells. It rarely infects CD4+ cells and is therefore unlikely to meet and mate with HIV.

Unfortunately, the other main branch of this family is only too relevant. It contains STLV-I and HTLV-I, both primarily attracted to CD4+ cells, just like SIV and HIV. The relationship of these simian and human tumor viruses is complex, so we should look first at their probable origin, then follow the two separately and connect them at a later stage.

One thing is crystal clear: STLV-I and HTLV-I, unlike SIV and HIV, entered the primate population long ago in Asia. According to genetic data, the oldest HTLV-I is from the southeastern Pacific. The oldest simian viruses are those of Indian and Indonesian macaques, like the rhesus, crab-eating, and pig-tailed macaques. Since the Barbary ape is negative for STLV, the virus did not come from Africa. Either STLV never infected this African ancestor of the entire macaque family or, less likely, it once did and then became extinct in Africa. The data suggest that the Asian macaques gave the virus to the humans now living in the southeastern Pacific. This seems impossible since Polynesian and Melanesian people live on islands never populated by monkeys. The only answer is that their ancestors and those of the macaques once shared an Asian habitat. In that primeval place, both the monkeys and the humans were infected by an ancestral STLV-I or HTLV-I. They subsequently found themselves, for whatever reason, in strictly separate habitats: the infected monkeys on the large islands of Indonesia, Java, Sumatra, and Borneo; the infected humans on Papua New Guinea, the Solomon Islands, Banks Islands, Torres Islands, and Australia. The Polynesian and Melanesian peoples are known to have traveled incredible distances in small boats.

From the primeval habitat, some macaques apparently took STLV to Japan. This event can be traced to a time when *Macaca fascicularis* and *Macaca fuscata* were the same species, and macaques covered all Japanese islands except Hokkaido. In the same period, some humans must have brought HTLV-I to Okinawa, and then to Hokkaido. (Since monkeys have never lived on Hokkaido, the human virus there must have been acquired from other humans. It could not have passed to humans from monkeys.) These or other Asians with HTLV-I much later crossed the Bering Sea, which explains the presence of this virus among today's Alaskan Eskimos and Amerindians.

When HTLV-II came to the Americas, it seems to have taken the same route as HTLV-I, but from Mongolia and not the Sunda Strait. As discussed below, human population movements are the only way to explain the finding of HTLV-I in ancient populations of both Japan and the Americas, and HTLV-II among both Mongolians and northern Amerindians.

Thousands of years after these events, STLV-I appears to have traveled to East Africa from its Asian homeland. It seems to have gone west long before HTLV because we see STLV in just about every monkey species inhabiting northeastern African countries like Ethiopia (baboons and grivets) and southeastern countries like Tanzania and Kenya (baboons and vervets). However, following that path, we rarely see HTLV in neighboring humans. This suggests that only after STLV infection reached monkeys in countries like the Central African Republic and Zaire (blue monkeys, redtail monkeys, and tantalus monkeys) and West African countries like Senegal, Sierra Leone, and Liberia (patas, sabaeus monkeys) did chimpanzees finally get the virus and pass it to humans as HTLV.

Of course, though all types of STLV and HTLV arose in Asia and fanned out from there, their hosts originally came from Africa with the great prehistoric migrations. Little is known about the prehistoric movements of monkeys. We do not know whether they traveled alone or were mainly brought by humans as pets or food. But ancient human migration patterns can be quite well reconstructed based on traits shared by people in different parts of the world. These traits can be genotypic or phenotypic. The genotype of any living thing is the genetic blueprint contained in its genome. The phenotype is the physical expression of that blueprint: how the creature looks and functions. The most useful indicators are traits that depend on more than one gene and are minimally skewed by environmental factors.

Migrations of People: Sundadonts and Sinodonts

To place the development of given traits (and the migration of people with these traits) on an accurate time scale, one must study them in people living at different points on the scale. Ideally, one compares modern people with people of ancient times. Since genetic traits are based on DNA evidence (like the evolution of mitochondrial DNA), and such evidence from ancient human remains is very unreliable, researchers focus on modern DNA evidence. Extrapolating from this, they must reconstruct the history of traits based on the assumption that they evolved at a constant rate, and can thus be used as a molecular clock. But this is just an assumption, so genetic evidence must be considered indirect or circumstantial.

A more direct alternative is the phenotypic evidence provided by dental anthropology. Of all physical remains, teeth are most plentiful and tend to last longest, so they can serve as an evolutionary yardstick for anthropologists, archaeologists, and other scientists. Christy Turner, a professor of anthropology at Arizona State University, has been able to paint a picture of the great prehistoric migrations based on the comparison of teeth of ancient and living populations. Based on variable features of teeth like bumps, ridges, and grooves, he has divided the Asian-Pacific peoples into Sundadonts and Sinodonts. Both groups are generally recognized as members of the Mongoloid race, but their teeth set them apart. According to Turner, the Sundadonts are the older population, descended from African people who migrated from Africa to the Sunda Shelf. These were the people who shared the primeval habitat with the Asian macaques, then went to Japan, the Pacific, and other points.

The Sunda Shelf is a vast continental plain that connects island and mainland Southeast Asia. It was dry land twenty thousand years ago, when the sea level was much lower than today. By about twelve thousand years ago, the sea had risen and separated the mainland from the Indonesian Archipelago, Japan, and other Southeast Asian islands. This gradually isolated the Sundadonts in the archipelago from those who had migrated to Okinawa and Hokkaido. We know this from finding Sundadont dental patterns in seventeen-thousand-year-old Minatogawa skeletons on the island of Okinawa, indicating that these people settled there before the waters rose. The Ryukyuan people of Okinawa and the Ainu of Hokkaido are Sundadonts. The rest of the Japanese people—including those of Kyushu—are Sinodonts.

Meanwhile, some Sundadonts of Indonesia gradually moved north as two separate nomad populations (Figure 9.3). One migrated along the coast of China. The other headed into the interior of China. Some of the coastal group sailed out to Polynesia and Melanesia about 1000 B.C. In Mongolia and the north of China, the interior Sundadonts evolved into Sinodonts while spreading in various directions. This happened sometime after the sea rose (18,000–13,000 B.C.) and before the Sinodont pattern became well established in northern China (c. 9000 B.C.). About two millennia ago, Sinodonts crossed from southern China to Japan to form the modern Japanese population.

Even earlier, perhaps 10,000 B.C., some of the interior Sinodonts traveled north from Mongolia to Siberia and across to Alaska. Over the next few thousand years, these Sinodonts flowed down over the Americas in three main waves. The first wave included ancestors of all the Amerindians of South America and many of North America. The second included the ancestors of the Aleuts and the Eskimos in the far north of North America. The last wave included the ancestors of the Navaho and Apache peoples and the Amerindians of British Columbia and the Alaskan interior.

This ancient migration pattern so closely resembles the ancient history of the HTLVs that we might safely assume that, in origin, HTLV-I is a Sundadont virus and HTLV-II is a Sinodont virus. HTLV-I was the virus passed to a Sundadont by a macaque (or vice versa) in their common habitat before Japan became isolated. Some Sundadonts took the virus to Australia and Papua New Guinea, which explains why we see it there today. Others

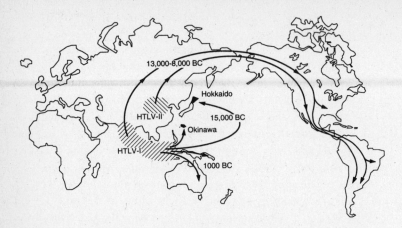

Figure 9.3   Travels and distribution of human T-cell leukemia viruses type I and II. *Hatching shows earliest habitats of HTLV-1 and HTLV-II, from which these retroviruses migrated with humans between 15,000 and 1,000* B.C. *HTLV-I, the oldest of the two, is most widespread in Asia and the oceanic area. The Americas are dominated by HTLV-II, but HTLV-I also was imported in ancient and modern times.* (Asher et al. 1988; Gessain, Gallo, and Franchini 1992; Ishida et al. 1985.)

took it to Okinawa and Hokkaido, and their subsequent isolation explains why HTLV-I is seen in the descendants of the most ancient Japanese: the Ryukyuan and the Ainu. Some Sundadonts of Indonesia later took the virus to the small islands of Polynesia and Melanesia.

Of the Mongolian and northern China Sundadonts, who evolved into Sinodonts and migrated to the Americas, only a few carried HTLV-I. We find traces of it today among descendants of the second and third wave: the Alaskan Eskimos and the Amerindians of British Columbia. Most Sinodonts carried HTLV-II, which they brought to America in their first wave of migration. This explains the presence of HTLV-II among the so-called indigenous people of South America. (Obviously, indigenous is in the eye of the beholder. If you go back far enough, hardly anybody is indigenous.) But what explains the HTLV-II we see today in Africa among the Zairian forest people? Since the Sinodonts acquired this virus long after they had left Africa, it can only appear there now because of a more recent transfer.

More important to our story is the older transfer to Africa of STLV and HTLV-I. How and when did STLV get there? Why do we find two distinct groups of HTLV-I strains in neighboring parts of West Africa? Why does one group resemble Kyushu-like strains that cause adult T-cell leukemia? Why do we find this same type of HTLV-I in the southern United States, the Caribbean, and the northeastern coast of South America?

The genetic evidence shows that STLV-I came to East Africa with macaques from India or Indonesia. These animals could have wandered back to their prehistoric homeland. More likely they were brought by sailors who took them aboard as pets and in some cases left them behind. From the tenth to the sixteenth century, Indonesian sailors frequented the East African coasts, as did Arab and Indian traders. They brought goods from the whole of Asia, including China. In the sixteenth century, the Portuguese acquired strongholds on the East African coast and opened a trade route to Asia and their main Asian trading capital, Malacca, in the Malay Peninsula. Any of these seafaring traders could have introduced STLV-I into Africa sometime after the tenth century. The virus then moved slowly westward across Africa, leaving humans relatively untouched until it became adapted to chimpanzees. This adaptation sufficiently lowered the barrier between apes and humans to allow cross-species transmission. Humans were then infected by HTLV-I in the interior of Zaire, where the virus has largely remained.

The idea that this virus passed to humans from monkeys or apes was recently bolstered by analysis of a strain isolated from one of the local forest people. His strain, which appears to resemble others among his people, has been shown to be a first-generation descendant of a grivet strain. In this man, perhaps bitten by a grivet, an STLV-I strain has set up housekeeping in its first human host. It has become HTLV-I by the same process that SIV sm becomes HIV-2.

Contribution of the Slave Trade

Far away, on the coast of Zaire and in West Africa, there is another group of HTLV-I strains with an entirely different history. They did not come from the humans of interior Zaire or from monkeys anywhere in Africa, not even from monkeys of West Africa. These West African viruses are closer to

HTLV-I strains of the Kyushu type. They were spread by the economic expansion of European countries in the sixteenth and seventeenth centuries and its most infamous consequence: the African slave trade.

In the sixteenth century the Portuguese sought to bypass Muslim North Africa and gain direct access to the gold in sub-Saharan West Africa. They built Elmina, Axim, and other fortresses at the Gold Coast in Ghana. Later, when they developed sugar plantations on the nearby islands of Príncipe and São Tomé, they initiated a limited slave trade. Slaves from Senegal and the Gambia were transported to farms and plantations in southern Spain and Portugal; slaves from the Niger delta and the Zaire river went to the African island plantations. Meanwhile, the Spaniards were opening up the transatlantic route to the Caribbean and the Americas. They, too, engaged in limited slave trade (Figure 9.4).

Gallo has argued on several occasions that the Portuguese traders formed the link between strains on Kyushu and related strains in Africa, the Caribbean, and the Americas. But another explanation seems more likely. The Portuguese controlled the slave trade for only a short period, and not during its peak. They never controlled the plantations in the Caribbean, which received the largest share of slaves. Also, their control of trade with Kyushu and Malacca was of short duration. This was because, early in the seventeenth century, both they and the Spanish ran into fierce competition, mainly from one small European country: the Netherlands. In 1637, about 150 years after the Portuguese built Elmina, the Dutch seized it and, in 1642, put a complete end to the Portuguese presence on the Gold Coast by taking Axim. The Dutch kept these and other West African strongholds till the late nineteenth century.

At about the same time that the Portuguese lost supremacy over the Gold Coast, the Spanish lost their hold in the Caribbean and the South American coastlands. The Caribbean islands were taken over by French, English, Danish, and the Dutch. By 1640, very labor-intensive plantations for sugar and tobacco had been established in Brazil and the Caribbean, creating an enormous demand for manpower. The British, French, and Dutch traders were very willing to satisfy this demand. The number of slaves transported rose from a few thousand a year in the sixteenth century to about twenty thousand a year in the seventeenth century, and finally to about one hundred thousand a year in the eighteenth century. The numbers declined drastically in the nineteenth century, and the slave trade stopped by the 1880s.

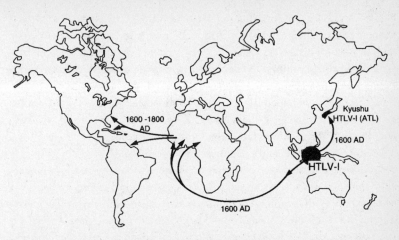

Figure 9.4   Origin of HTLV-I and its modern migration. *This ancient Sundadont virus probably passed to humans from monkeys in Southeast Asia when the two species shared a primeval habitat. From 1600 to 1800, European colonialism and trade took disease-causing strains from Kyushu to West Africa and the Caribbean.* (Boxer 1930; Gallo et al. 1986; van Lier 1949; Lewis 1995; Stellingwerff 1983.)

So there are three contenders for the dubious honor of dispersing HTLV-I and adult T-cell leukemia: the French, the English, and the Dutch. The history of trade with Japan reveals the last piece of the puzzle. By 1641 the Dutch dominated trade between Europe and the East. They had built a strong trading post in Batavia on the Indonesian island of Java, and in 1641 forces of the United Netherlands East Indies Company took over the Portuguese fortress of Malacca. By that time the Dutch West Indies Company controlled a large part of the slave trade to the West Indies. In Japan the Dutch again competed with the Portuguese, who traded at Nagasaki and several other ports of Kyushu from 1550 onward. In 1623, political unrest and perhaps fear of European invasion caused the Japanese to expel the Spanish Jesuits. In that same year they put the Portuguese under house arrest, which continued until 1636, when all Portuguese (numbering 287) were moved to the artificial island of Deshima in Nagasaki Harbor. That fall, the Portuguese left Japan forever, and Japan began the Sakoku, or "closed country," era that lasted until 1853.

Of all the European nations, only the Dutch were allowed to have a trading post on Japanese soil and to trade with the Japanese during that long era. The Dutch had been in Japan since 1600, despite several Portuguese and Jesuit efforts to expel them. However, from 1641 onward, the Dutch were pretty much confined to Deshima, left five years earlier by the Portuguese. A fan-shaped island in the harbor, it was close to the only other foreign enclave: Juzenji Mura of the Chinese traders. On Deshima, a very small island, about twenty Dutchmen lived year-round.

According to a Japanese publication from 1708 (*Kwai-Tsusho-Ko*, by Nishikawa Joken of Kyoto), the Dutch imported both large and small monkeys into Japan. One of the so-called Nagasaki prints, made by Hayashi Shihei in 1782, has an inscription describing Dutch ships with black people aboard. Including Africans and dark-skinned Indonesians, they were imported for use as servants to the Dutch. The Japanese called them *swardo jongo* from Dutch *zwarte jongen*, black boys.

No Dutch women were allowed in Japan, and any Japanese woman who married a Dutchman was sent to Holland. However, prostitutes regularly visited Deshima from Nagasaki's red-light district, Maruyama. In fact, special prostitutes assigned to the Dutch, called *orandayuki,* or visitors of the Dutch, sometimes remained a week at a time with their clients in Deshima. The many children that were born of Dutch men and these women (or female servants) were considered Japanese. They were raised as Japanese and often kept away from their fathers. Never were they allowed to leave Japan with their fathers. One wonders if modern Japanese who are positive for HTLV-1 are all descended from these children.

All this ancient and modern history is anchored at many points by genetic data. As we have said, the oldest HTLV-1 is the virus of the Sundadonts in the Indonesian archipelago. Thousands of years ago, some strains were taken to Japanese islands, where they evolved on their own. The rest circulated among the peoples of Indonesia, also evolving on their own. Then, in the last few hundred years, trade brought one of the Indonesian strains to Kyushu in Japan. Perhaps it was passed to a Dutch man by a prostitute in Batavia, Malacca, or southern India (where Kyushu-type viruses also circulate) or by an Indonesian servant woman. The Dutch man could then have passed it to a Japanese prostitute. Or perhaps a woman of Kyushu had relations with an Indonesian manservant of the Dutch. Having entered the Kyushu population, this HTLV-I was passed on by mother-to-infant transmission, remaining confined to the south of Kyushu and sometimes causing adult T-cell leukemia.

Meanwhile, because of the slave trade, this same virus reached West Africans (Figure 9.4). Perhaps a Dutch trader who had spent time on Deshima came to West Africa and had relations with a woman there. Apparently, the virus became better and better adapted to vaginal transmission as it passaged through the local people of West Africa. When many went as slaves to the plantations of the southern United States, the Caribbean, and the northeastern coast of South America, they brought HTLV-I of the Kyushu type. In just a few hundred years the virus had traveled this far because of increased host movement in many parts of the world. European colonialism and commerce brought the AIDS viruses out of the African rain forest and the tumor viruses out of Asia.

When HIV emerged, two groups of HTLV-I were already settled in Africa, first in interior Zaire and later in West Africa. In the Americas and Asia as well, HTLV-I infections predated the HIV influx of this century. On the other hand, it appears that SIV predated STLV in Africa. In any case, these two families of viruses have waited a long time to meet. But in the present era of mobility and changing conditions, SIV and STLV now cocirculate among African monkeys, and HTLV and HIV cocirculate among people in Africa and the Americas. The two families have finally aligned their hosts, target cells, and modes of transmission so that they can infect the very same cell. Double infections have already been seen in monkeys and humans. Usually they cause no disease, but two very sick African green monkeys have shown their potential.

It is a only matter of time until recombinants emerge with new properties inherited from both parent viruses. Most new properties will do us no harm; some will harm the viruses. But in the random shuffling of genes, some dangerous offspring could well appear: retroviruses with improved infectivity; retroviruses that cause AIDS epidemics in African monkeys; or retroviruses that cause both AIDS and cancers.

10

Viral Sex and AIDS: Response to Instability

AIDS epidemics are unique to retroviruses but not to just one kind of retrovirus. AIDS in humans is caused by three lentiviruses (HIV-0, HIV-1, and HIV-2), which we have traced back to innocent viruses in the jungles of Africa. But AIDS in cats is caused by a very different type of retrovirus (FeLV), which does most harm when working with another (FIV). Such collaboration between retroviruses has been spotted in humans and monkeys. Even if they cause no disease, these double infections are a threat in their potential for recombinants. Sex between lentiviruses and other retroviruses appears to be the main way they obtain new features, and these features can be dangerous.

We have argued that two harmless viruses can recombine to cross species, and that in some cases this process results in AIDS. Can we find an example that offers us both parents for study? The recombinant HIV-1E will not do because we cannot know if both parents were harmless at their mating, and one parent has completely disappeared. Nor will the recombinant sabaeus SIV agm serve our purposes. Both its parents were apparently harmless but, here again, one is no longer available.

The example we need caused a nearly forgotten epidemic among captive macaques that began about 1970. Few people noticed this epidemic of AIDS-like disease, which was overshadowed by the human and monkey AIDS epidemics of the early 1980s. Few now refer to it, since its agent is totally unrelated to SIV or HIV. But that epidemic is of utmost relevance to our understanding of the true nature of AIDS in humans. Its agent is harmless to its one natural host, a unique and little known species of African monkey. The virus actually originated in rodents and picked up an envelope in monkeys to form a recombinant that causes AIDS in unaccustomed hosts. The story of this monkey AIDS virus is the story of the human AIDS viruses, only a little more complete.

About a year before captive macaques were infected by the SIV of sooty mangabeys, the California Primate Research Center (CPRC) reported a series of four outbreaks of AIDS-like disease in rhesus macaques in the *Lancet* (Henrickson, 1983). The first outbreak had occurred between 1969 and 1975, affecting forty-two animals. The second occurred in the early 1970s in a group of fifty-four macaques, of which forty-four died between 1976 and 1978. The third started in 1976 and lasted until 1981, when all diseased animals were removed from their outdoor enclosure, known as corral 1. This left eight healthy juvenile females, to which fifty-six healthy macaques were added in August 1981, making a total of sixty four. By the time the *Lancet* report appeared, twenty-four of those sixty-four animals had died during the fourth and final outbreak.

The authors suggested that immune suppression due to a common cause linked the whole series. Their findings clearly pointed to a transmissible agent. In the fourth outbreak this agent had apparently been introduced by one animal, a rhesus macaque born April 1978 in corral 1. When she was four months old, her mother died during the third outbreak, so she was moved to the CPRC nursery and young infant ward. By 1981, when taken back to the corral, she had infected no animals in the nursery because of separate caging. But in the young infant ward up to five animals share space, and two of her cage-mates died of AIDS. At this point the culprit—still apparently healthy and unsuspected—was moved to an outdoor cage. She moved several times before finally returning to corral 1 among the fifty-six newcomers who joined the eight survivors of the third outbreak. By the time her virus had killed twenty-four of that group, it had killed thirty-four animals in all. Looking back, it was seen that she had killed animals each time she moved to a new cage. Virus isolation yielded a retrovirus from her saliva, blood, and urine.

When saliva of this monkey was injected into the bloodstream of two healthy juvenile rhesus macaques, both were infected by her virus and both developed AIDS. However, the infecting monkey was found negative for both SIV and STLV-1, as were the two experimentally infected animals. So an unknown retrovirus was suspected. In the spring of 1984 it was identified by groups from the California and Washington primate centers. Preston Marx, then at CPRC, claimed in March that it was a D-type retrovirus. A month later Stromberg and Benveniste of the National Cancer Institute, in collaboration with the Washington people, confirmed his claim. The new agent was called *simian retrovirus* (SRV) (Figures 10.1 and 10.2).

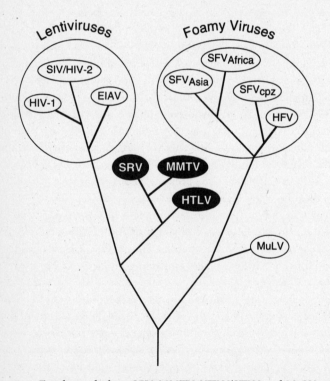

Figure 10.1   *Family tree linking SRV, MMTV, HTLV/STLV, and MuLV to main branches of lentiviruses and foamy viruses.* (Herchenröder et al. 1994; Mergia et al. 1990; Schweizer and Neumann-Maefelin 1995; Bieniasz et al. 1995.)

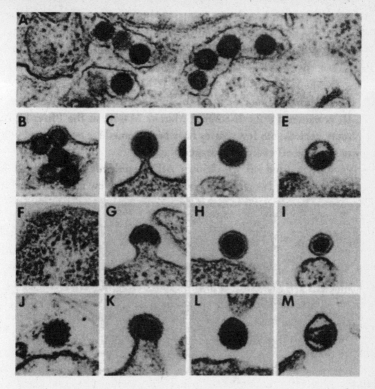

Figure 10.2 **Morphology of retrovirus types**. *Row one, A-type particles; row two, B-type (MMTV); row three, C-type (MuLV and BAEV); row four, D-type (MPMV and SRV). Electron micrographs by Gonda et al., 1989.*

The strain identified at the CPRC was soon designated SRV-1 after another member of the family was identified, again by Marx. This second virus, SRV-2, was found at primate centers of Washington and Oregon. Then SRV-3 was found at a primate center in Wisconsin. It was recently joined by SRV-4 at the primate center of the University of California, Berkeley, and SRV-5 at the center in Beijing, China.

The whole family infects macaque species, and some strains cause not only the usual opportunistic infections but retroperitoneal fibromatosis. Strongly associated with SRV-2, this invariably fatal disease was first noticed at the Washington primate center in the mid-1970s. It involves the formation of fibromatous tissue that gradually fills the abdominal cavity,

encircling the intestines and encapsulating the liver, the spleen, and the
kidneys. It ultimately strangles and blocks all functions of these organs,
thereby killing the monkey. The virus causing this dreadful disease was not
entirely new. SRVs are variants of Mason-Pfizer monkey virus (MPMV),
the first D-type retrovirus to be discovered. MPMV was isolated in 1969
from the mammary tumor of a rhesus monkey and reported in August
1970. (It is named for its discoverer, Marcus Mason, at the Pfizer Company. Many bacteria but few viruses have been named for people, and viral
eponyms are now officially discouraged.)

SRVs have caused all the known AIDS epidemics among captive
macaques, except for two: the 1984 outbreak at the New England Primate
Center (see Chapter 6) and one at the Louisiana Delta Primate Center,
both caused by SIV. In vitro, SRV and MPMV can infect cell lines of humans, mink, bats, monkeys, and cats, indicating their promiscuity in terms
of species. They are also promiscuous in their preferred cell type. They
multiply primarily in fibroblasts, which are connective tissue cells that can
form collagen. They also thrive in the lymphocytes of baboon and rhesus
monkeys and in human B- and T-cell lines.

How SRVs spread was at first a mystery. The fact that the virus was isolated from blood, urine, saliva, breast milk, tears, and vaginal secretions did
not help. So the California group of Marx and Gardner designed a very effective experiment to address this issue. They reconfigured corral 1, site of
the third and fourth SRV outbreaks, to include two enclosures separated by
a ten-foot buffer zone that prevented direct physical contact between the
animals in the two enclosures. Into one enclosure they put fifty-three
macaques of the group that had suffered from AIDS, plus twenty-three
healthy juveniles from a troop never touched by SIV, SRV, or AIDS. Other
juveniles from the same healthy troop were put, by themselves, in the second enclosure.

The results were dramatic. Of juveniles in direct contact with the sick
monkeys, 83 percent (nineteen of twenty-three) died within the year. No
AIDS occurred in the group without physical contact, so apparently the
virus was not carried by air. Nor was it carried by bites from insects that
might have traveled between the groups. Clearly, direct physical contact
was needed to acquire the causative agent of this form of AIDS—but what
kind of contact? Transmission by air or insects had been eliminated, but
that left intrauterine and perinatal transmission, transmission through ingestion of breast milk, transmission by licking, biting, and grooming, and

transmission by sex. So the data were analyzed for clues based on the age distribution of infection and disease among different monkey groups.

During the 2.5-year follow-up period, not only did nineteen of the newly introduced juveniles die, but also twenty-six monkeys already living in the enclosure. However, the new juveniles were the first to die from AIDS; in fact, they accounted for all deaths of the first year. The resident juveniles were the next victims, most of them dying in the second year of the experiment. Last of all, a few resident infants died. Over the whole time, resident adults were relatively spared. These differences seen among distinct age groups can be explained either by variation in exposure to infection or by variation in disease development related to host age at the time of infection.

The rare and late development of disease among newborns shows that perinatal infection by SRV is uncommon. The lower disease rate among adults, compared with juveniles, suggests that developing animals are much more vulnerable to SRV infection than mature animals. It suggests transmission by juvenile activities like playful grooming or biting instead of adult activities like sex.

The data confirmed that SRV-1 could cause AIDS not only experimentally but in natural circumstances. About 85 percent of animals in the diseased enclosure were infected with SRV-1, yet not even 5 percent were infected with SIV or STLV-1. In the healthy enclosure, no SRV-1 could be found. The study also demonstrated that a buffer zone of only ten feet was sufficient quarantine against infection by this virus. The same is surely also true for SIV, HIV, and the tumor viruses since, like SRV, they require direct contact. They must be applied directly to mucosal surfaces by sexual activity; or they must encounter circulating blood cells through ingestion (as in breast-feeding) or a skin break.

But what would make the newly introduced juveniles more SRV-susceptible than resident juveniles, infants, and adults? This is easily explained and may have benefits for us. The point is that the new juveniles were born to non-SRV-infected mothers, whereas the resident juveniles were born to SRV-infected mothers. SRV infection induces a virus-neutralizing or protective antibody response, particularly in healthy carriers of the virus. When the carrier is pregnant, these antibodies leak through the placenta to the fetus. After birth they are detectable for more than a year, and the infant acquires additional SRV antibodies with its mother's milk. Despite all these circulating antibodies, infants are readily infected by SRV, probably by the saliva of peers or parents. However, SRV antibodies seem to delay the onset of disease. Juveniles born to uninfected mothers, who get no SRV antibodies, do not necessarily get infected sooner, but they definitely get sick much sooner than those born to infected mothers.

These observations demonstrate an intriguing mechanism that does not protect against infection but protects against—or postpones—disease. To supply such protection, SRV antibodies could be injected by vaccination. A less direct approach would be to inject antigens from the SRV envelope that would stimulate an immune response. The host would then manufacture its own extra SRV antibodies. They might not prevent infection but, like those acquired from infected mothers, might very well postpone or prevent disease.

However, though this might work with SRV, it might not work with SIV or HIV. After all, newborns are infected, not protected, by HIV-infected mothers. They acquire the virus both during delivery and from breast milk, with a high rate of progression to AIDS in both cases. The difference is that the saliva route of infection is major for SRV infection (and viruses like FeLV of cats) but minor or nonexistent for infection with SIV or HIV. Conversely, the anal or vaginal route of infection is major for SIV and HIV but very minor for SRV. Thus we see no SIV or HIV in juveniles (i.e., those not sexually mature or active), the very group most vulnerable to SRV infection.

Still, the disease postponement mechanism may help us with SIV/HIV. If it could be used to reduce the load just when the virus is establishing infection, it might diminish its damaging effects. Admittedly, virus load seems to play a different role in these two retrovirus families. The load, or *quantity*, of virus is the main factor in immunosuppression by SIV and HIV. For SRV the main factor is the *quality* of the virus: the way the SRV envelope interacts with the host immune system. For both virus families, however, both quantitative and qualitative aspects have influence. For both families, it matters how much virus is circulating. More virus is not a good sign in either case.

Work of our own group and that of the Dutch Primate Center has clearly shown that although vaccination of chimpanzees with the HIV envelope does not prevent infection, it definitely lowers the virus load at the time of infection. In some individuals the load becomes undetectable. Of course, infected chimpanzees under natural conditions are not susceptible to disease regardless of virus load. However, work with susceptible monkeys has shown that disease is postponed in animals injected with antibodies from macaques that are SIV-infected but asymtomatic long term. So a vaccine that can lower virus load in a new host might do a lot of good even if it cannot prevent infection.

Where did SRV come from? It turns out to be endemic in some primate centers and not in others. Within affected primate centers, some colonies have very high infection rates and others have no infection whatsoever. When SRV occurs, it affects all kinds of macaques imported from many locations in Asia, indicating that Asian macaques in general are very susceptible to SRV infection. Macaques from Indonesia (tonkeana, crab-eating, and celebes crested macaques), India (rhesus macaques), China (Taiwanese rock macaques), and Japan (Japanese macaques) all have been shown to be infected in captivity.

However, SRV is not an Asian virus. An extensive survey was done by Linda Löwenstine from the CPRC, where the whole SRV story started. At six US zoos, Löwenstine tested all major groups of Old World monkeys and apes from both Asia and Africa. Her most striking finding was that only one Indonesian crab-eating macaque out of about one hundred individuals and nine macaque species was infected with SRV. This argues that SRV is not endemic in Asian feral macaques. The Asian apes and colobine monkeys she studied were also SRV-negative, which suggests that no Asian monkeys are infected in the wild; they are vulnerable only when exposed in affected primate centers. Löwenstine then tested African monkeys but found virtually no sign of SRV. The chimpanzees and gorillas she tested were negative, as were the mandrills and other baboons, mangabeys, and guenons, including all four subspecies of African green monkeys.

Löwenstine found SRV abundantly present in only one African monkey species: the talapoin monkey of West Africa (Figure 10.3). She detected the virus in 67 percent of the fifteen talapoins she tested at US zoos. Of course, like the macaques who acquired SRV in primate centers, these talapoins might have acquired SRV in the zoos. Was SRV really a talapoin virus circulating among talapoins in their natural African surrounding? The answer is yes. Desrosiers of the New England Primate Center tested talapoins recently captured in Africa and held in quarantine by a US primate importer. Like Löwenstine, he found the majority positive for SRV. But he found no SRV in monkeys that share their native habitat: wild-

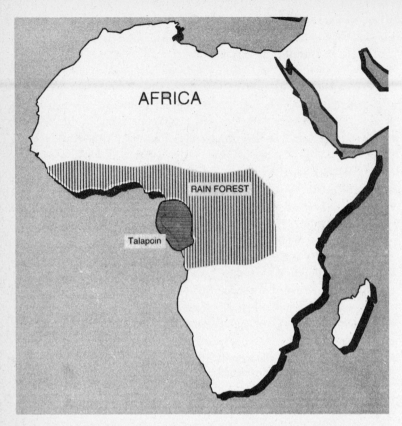

Figure 10.3 **Location of talapoins in the central African rain forest.**
(Haltenorth 1977.)

caught guenons, chimpanzees, and baboons. So SRV apparently is a talapoin virus that infects talapoins under natural conditions but none of
their neighbors.

The talapoin monkey is the smallest of all African primates, about the
size of a large squirrel. At one time it was considered a separate genus,
Miopithecus, but more recent primatologists have lumped it with guenons
(*Cercopithecus*). However, unlike guenons, talapoin females show sexual
swelling, and our own genetic data argue that this monkey is not a guenon.
Biologists have long agreed that it is not one of the Papionini tribe, given its

higher chromosome number. Talapoins live at the edges of the western equatorial rain forest in southwestern Cameroon, Gabon, and Congo. They love water, are renowned swimmers, and generally sleep on low branches overhanging water. They often live close to villages but are not kept as pets. They are usually seen as pesky raiders of crops and food storage areas.

The origin of their virus, SRV, is a mystery since they are its only host in Africa and perhaps in the whole world. SRV is clearly one of the rarest of primate retroviruses, if not the rarest. It is an innocent virus in its usual host but can readily cause AIDS in certain other hosts. Probably it has not spread to other primates in the region because of low infectivity. The reason cannot be lack of opportunity, since talapoins have much more interaction with local monkeys and humans than, for example, the chimpanzee. Yet the talapoin virus has remained confined while the chimpanzee virus was passed to humans as HIV-0 and HIV-1.

Study of the genetic buildup of SRV reveals clues to its origin and relationships (Figures 10.1 and 10.2). Since retroviruses are distinguished by reverse transcriptase, they all have a gene that codes for this enzyme. The gene is highly conserved, so its tiny variations can reveal genetic relationships. These show that the closest relative of SRV is a B-type murine virus: mouse mammary tumor virus (MMTV). This retrovirus of mice usually lies dormant in the cell genome, passing from host to offspring with the genetic material. It is therefore considered endogenous, but under certain conditions it can be activated to produce exogenous particles, or virions. Exogenous or infectious viruses can spread from host to host, and are more often harmful than endogenous viruses. In the case of MMTV, its activation can cause breast cancer in its original host. Its virions can be transmitted in breast milk to offspring that may themselves develop breast cancer. Of course, the offspring also inherit the dormant endogenous MMTV.

SRV is an exogenous virus. It is not passed genetically among talapoins but spreads in saliva, causing harmless infections. The close relationship of this virus with MMTV is confirmed by all their genes except one. The SRV gene that codes for the viral envelope is not at all like its MMTV counterpart. This suggests that SRV is a recombinant with a mouse virus parent (from which it got most of its genes) and a primate virus parent (from which it got the envelope gene). The envelope of SRV looks very much like that of endogenous C-type retroviruses of primates, for example, the CPC-1 virus of colobus monkeys and BaEV of baboons and African green monkeys. For reasons explained in the next chapter, a B-type MMTV-like retrovirus needed a C-type envelope from a primate virus to create the D-type SRV. It needed this primate envelope so it could spread in primates.

SRV has not yet spread far, but we can tell it did not originate in the talapoin. So it has spread at least to this one species by the infectious route, probably through biting or licking the original host species. The animal in which SRV was born must have shared the talapoin habitat when the recombination event occurred. It may still live nearby, but SRV has not yet been isolated from any animal but talapoins. The virus may have died out in its original host, having found talapoins more comfortable.

The mystery animal was probably a primate that carries other D-type viruses. In the late 1970s, long before SRV was known to cause AIDS in monkeys, the Asian langur was found to harbor an endogenous D-type virus very similar to SRV. The langur is a monkey belonging to the Asian branch of the colobus monkeys. Endogenous D-type viruses related to the langur virus have also been found in African colobus monkeys and monkeys of the Papionini tribe like baboons. Talapoins have never lived with Asian colobines or African green monkeys, but they encounter certain African colobines. The black colobus (*Colobus satanas*) is a severely endangered monkey species whose only remaining habitat is in the western equatorial region roamed by talapoin monkeys. SRV has not been isolated from these animals, but so few have been available for testing that they cannot yet be ruled out as the original host (see Chapter 11).

Whatever the mystery animal, it harbored two endogenous viruses that mated and produced SRV. How could this unlikely event occur? As we know, endogenous retroviruses are found in the genome of every single cell of a given species. They originate when a virus infects an embryo in its earliest stage (before cell differentiation), and viral genes become a permanent part of the host germ line. When this has happened long ago, the endogenous retrovirus is often quite defective. Its gene function has been taken over by cellular machinery. Stretches of its DNA have been randomly deleted during cell division and host procreation.

But relatively new endogenous retroviruses—those recently introduced into the cellular genome—are often complete. Activation can cause them to generate complete virions that contain no cellular DNA but two strands of RNA (coding for the endogenous viral DNA). These virus particles can reproduce and are categorized according to what conditions they require. When the endovirus (or its virions) can reproduce only in cells of the same species, the virus is *ecotropic*. When reproduction can occur only in cells of a different species, the virus is *xenotropic*. When reproduction can occur either way, the virus is *polytropic*.

Now, if a host genome contains two endogenous viruses that happen to shed complete virions, these may infect a common cell in a common host. This is most likely their original host, but it could conceivably be some new individual of the same or different species. Having met, the two virions could mate and produce a recombinant, given nucleic acid stretches with sufficient homology to recombine.

Looking at SRV, we can speculate that a mouse (or other rodent) bit a black colobus (or other monkey) that was pregnant with a very early fetus. The mouse carried an endogenous B-type virus of mice, an MMTV-like virus that was polytropic or xenotropic. This B-type virus became endogenous to the monkey fetus, which had already inherited an endogenous C-type primate virus. Thus the genome of every cell in the fetus contained these two endogenous viruses. At some point the two endogenous viruses both shed virions. Both Asian and African colobines are known to shed endogenous C-type retroviruses (CPC-1), as are baboons and African green monkeys (BaEV). One of the two particles enters a cell and waits until the other arrives. Their mating produces SRV, a D-type virus with its backbone derived from the mouse virus and its envelope from the monkey virus.

The envelope may seem a small contribution, but the envelope genes largely determine the host range and also the virulence of a virus. In order to spread effectively, a virus must interact with a particular structure on the surface of its preferred host cells. This interaction, which admits the virus to the cell, is largely dependent on the viral envelope, that is, the network of envelope proteins that protrude from the viral coat.

For example, HIV and SIV can infect a certain cell type in a wide range of primates. They enter these cells through interaction of their viral envelope with the CD4 molecule on the cell surface, a receptor present only on certain immune cells in primates. A very similar molecule is found on mouse immune cells, but HIV and SIV cannot normally infect them. Even when recombinant DNA technology is used to plant the human CD4 receptor on the mouse cell surface, HIV and SIV cannot infect these cells. However, SIV and HIV can readily enter mouse immune cells that are already infected with endogenous mouse retroviruses. They do this by a short-term alternative to recombination: phenotypic mixing. By this process a virus temporarily extends its host range by putting on a disguise, in this case a better coat—a better set of envelope proteins.

How can this happen? When endogenous retroviruses reproduce, most of their reproductive functions are assumed by the cellular machinery. Cellular enzymes produce the envelope proteins that will stud the new virions. These proteins are expressed in the cell wall, where they wait until needed. When a new virion is ready to break out, it butts against the cell wall, a lipid bilayer. As it buds through, its genetic material is wrapped in a piece of the wall, which contains the envelope proteins. This piece of cell wall actually becomes the coat and envelope for the new virion.

Now, let us again visualize two different endogenous viruses as they reproduce simultaneously in the same cell. The cellular enzymes have made envelope proteins for both, which are waiting in the cell wall. When a new particle is wrapped, it gets an envelope with both kinds of proteins (Figure 10.4). Such an envelope can substantially change the interactive ability and host range of the new virion.

An experiment performed in 1990 by the Gallo group showed the amazing consequences of phenotypic mixing for HIV. The work involved two human T-cell lines that were identical, except that one had an endogenous mouse retrovirus and the other did not. HIV-1 reproduced slowly in the cells lacking the endogenous virus but like wildfire in cells containing the endovirus. So the presence of the endogenous retrovirus made the cells produce far more HIV-1 progeny. Not only that, but the progeny had envelopes combining HIV-1 proteins and mouse retrovirus proteins. They could infect not only the usual CD4+ cells but also CD4− skin cells, fibroblasts, and muscle cells. They could infect certain B cells previously considered nonsusceptible to HIV. They could infect primary CD8+ cells, that is, freshly sampled cells, not those immortalized in a cell line. (Remember that primary cells are generally less hospitable to growth than a corresponding cell line.) Even more striking, these phenotypically mixed variants could infect CD4+ cells of which the CD4 molecule was blocked by antibody. Obviously this new variant had vastly broadened its host cell range by means of the murine retrovirus envelope proteins in its coat. The promiscuous variant could even infect certain cells of nonprimates.

However, phenotypic mixing has its disadvantages. Unlike recombination, it is a limited and unstable process. The resulting viruses do not keep their new properties for long, certainly not into the next generation. And even while the new properties broaden their entry range, their infection of previously nonsusceptible cells is not very efficient. Phenotypic mixing is a transient improvement and may serve as a stepping-stone to recombina-

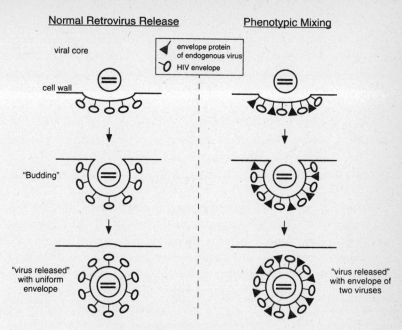

Figure 10.4 **Phenotypic mixing**. *Production of a normal HIV particle is shown at left. Production of phenotypically mixed HIV, at right, occurs when the host cell harbors an endogenous retrovirus. The cell machinery generates envelope proteins for both HIV and the endogenous virus. They are expressed on the cell surface. When HIV virions bud and break out, they are wrapped in cell wall studded with mixed proteins. This temporarily enables HIV to enter a greater range of cell types.*

tion. But viral sex and recombination are needed to engrave the new properties in the genetic code of the virus.

Does SRV Threaten Us?

The big question is whether recombination or phenotypic mixing could lead to SRV strains that cause AIDS in humans. The first requirement is a locale where SRV is circulating, which we have in the talapoin habitat. Humans live there and could therefore be infected by a talapoin. Or a human could be infected by one of these monkeys at a zoo or a primate center where SRV is endemic. It is well known that human cells, B-cell lines in particular, are extremely susceptible to SRV infection. Humans could presumably be infected in vivo if the virus in the saliva of a talapoin were to meet a human blood cell. A talapoin could easily bite an African villager or an animal care technician.

Fortunately for us, the efficiency of infection must be extremely low. Otherwise, with all this potential opportunity, local humans or monkeys would by now have been infected by SRV. Yet no SRV infections of Africans living in the talapoin habitat have been reported, nor have cases of SIV/HIV-negative AIDS been reported from these regions.

Since AIDS caused by SRV would have different indicator diseases than AIDS caused by SIV/HIV, have cases perhaps gone unnoticed? This is unlikely since, at least in macaques, a typical indicator is retroperitoneal fibromatosis—a very nasty disease that would not be overlooked if it caused an epidemic in humans or monkeys.

In 1991 the first report was published of SRV infection in an HIV-1-positive AIDS patient. This proved that SRV can infect humans but not that SRV is spreading in humans, since the case occurred under highly unusual conditions. In 1990 a thirty-two-year-old man was admitted to the University of Texas M. D. Anderson Cancer Center in Houston. HIV-1-positive and severely immunocompromised, the man was diagnosed with Burkitt's lymphoma, an aggressive tumor of the lymphoid organs. This B-cell lymphoma kept growing, and the man finally died from cancer at many locations in his body. Large syncytia were seen in the lymphoma tissue, so at first it was thought that the patient's HIV-1 strain was causing them. However, although aggressive HIV-1 strains are known to cause these multinucleated giant cells, they were seen here in B cells and not T cells, as would be expected with HIV-1.

The Texas researchers easily established three cell lines on this patient's B cells. (This was most likely easy because the B cells were immortalized by EBV, the type of herpesvirus that causes Burkitt's lymphoma.) When the cell lines were inspected by electron microscopy, virions were seen within the cells and in large numbers outside the cells. They looked much like the D-type MPMV or the closely related SRV. They were the right density to be a retrovirus. When purified and tested for reverse transcriptase, the virions revealed its activity. Their reverse transcriptase had all the features of that enzyme as observed in MPMV or SRV. The virus infected both B cells and T cells, which is typical of D-type retroviruses. No HIV or

HTLV was present in the cell lines, but SRV apparently was. Genetic characterization of the mystery retrovirus revealed strong homology to SRV and not to any other retrovirus family.

Of course, skeptics could argue that SRV was found because of a laboratory contamination. They could argue that SRV was not necessarily present in the primary, freshly sampled cells of the patient, on which the cell lines were founded. However, clarification was provided by polymerase chain reaction (PCR) analysis of the patient's bone marrow, which was full of SRV DNA. The putative SRV particles and DNA molecules could still be laboratory contaminations, so the Texas researchers also checked the patient for antibodies to SRV. They found them, as did an independent research group. This finally proved unequivocally that the patient was infected with SRV.

So we may be sure that this case truly represents the first reported human SRV infection. How the patient was infected is unknown. He could have acquired the infection before or after he got HIV and AIDS. The most realistic conclusion is that he acquired SRV as an opportunistic infection because HIV had compromised his ability to fight off infections. It is unlikely that he was infected in Cameroon or Gabon, so he probably met the virus at a zoo or a primate center. All around, the case was a rare and unlikely event. It proves that human cells are susceptible to SRV not only in vitro but in vivo, but only when the time and place are exactly right.

At this point SRV lacks the characteristics needed for efficient human infection. Its story nevertheless tells us a lot about retrovirus history and behavior. It shows that recombination between retroviruses can produce a new virus able not only to cross species barriers but to spread in the new species. An endogenous B-type mouse retrovirus and an endogenous C-type monkey retrovirus delivered the ingredients for a whole new class of viruses: the D-type retroviruses.

This event no doubt took place hundreds of thousands of years ago. For all that time, or at least for millennia, these D-type retroviruses circulated in a single species in Africa without infecting any other primate, human or nonhuman. Apparently, enough talapoins were available for SRV to spread its genes without being forced to jump and adapt to a less suitable host. Indeed, talapoins are abundantly present in the equatorial rain forest. They are not endangered at all.

Only when the virus went with its host to a new environment (US zoos or primate centers) was it so close to susceptible species that infection could occur. Because these new hosts were less suitable, the virus had to adapt, thus causing AIDS. Unlike HIV, it did not adapt by increasing its production and virus load. Most likely the new host was susceptible (through some mechanism as yet unknown) to the immunosuppressive effects of certain parts of the SRV envelope.

This story again shows the impact of human interference on animal environments. SRV is unlikely to give us AIDS unless we are caged with SRV-infected macaques or talapoins, an unlikely scenario. But could instability induce a similar sequence of events in a natural habitat shared by two retrovirus hosts?

11

Retrovirus Survival: The Human Threat

The SRV story shows how a retrovirus can change and spread in new species, causing disease when it was previously harmless. The story also shows that a retrovirus generally stays in its natural host species, causing little or no harm, as long as that species is widely available. As long as talapoin monkeys stay in the western equatorial rain forest, for example, SRV appears not to infect other susceptible species nearby. It enters such hosts only rarely and with insufficient persistence to establish itself. SRV and its talapoin host are mutually adapted.

Retroviral movement appears to be largely a function of environmental instability since the main force for retrovirus survival is adaptation to environmental change. Such change may concern the microenvironment of a single host or the macroenvironment of the host community, or a combination of both. The process seems to start at the macro level, where the main factor is the availability of susceptible hosts. After all, if an accustomed host is decimated, a virus dies with the host unless it happens to gain a foothold in a new species. The new host must be susceptible and close at hand, especially if close contact is needed for transmission.

These dynamics are entirely random and take place over many virus generations. In the case of chimpanzee SIV (SIV cpz), we can infer that this virus passed to humans—but not often or persistently—long before chimpanzees were ever endangered. Passage occurred simply because of opportunity. Now and then a chimpanzee bit a hunter and left a small population of SIV in a human host. Perhaps at first SIV cpz replicated poorly in humans, so such a population usually failed to cause infection. But now and then an odd strain would gain a foothold due to chance advantages in its makeup or circumstances. It infected a hospitable cell and produced progeny in the hunter or in someone to whom he passed bodily fluids. Of that progeny, the odd strain or two survived and in turn produced progeny in which a few survived, and so on. Eventually, after many virus generations and passages from human to human, a virus population evolved in which the majority could survive in humans. That is, the majority could infect and reproduce in humans, and only the odd ones could not. The latter became the minority because they did not survive. They continue to die—or reproduce weakly—whenever they appear.

At this point we say that "the virus has adapted," which seems to imply viral determination, but viruses cannot determine anything. They simply do or do not survive. Natural selection favors some, based on their chance advantages, while eliminating others. It sifts out the losers and leaves the winners, in a continual process that can always turn, sharply or gradually, in a different direction. An environmental change, such as natural disaster or new competition, can undermine and ultimately unseat the most long-standing winner, as occurred with the dinosaurs.

Many human-to-human passages were no doubt needed before chimpanzee SIV evolved into HIV-0 and HIV-1. Only when conditions were optimal for their dissemination among humans did HIV-0 and HIV-1 become relatively stable viral populations with a genetic makeup readily distinguishable from the chimpanzee SIV. Their evolution as human viruses began in the nineteenth century when human–chimpanzee contact began to increase. Subjected to more hunting and disturbance of food sources, chimpanzees eventually became endangered. Chimpanzee SIV was equally endangered (albeit oblivious) but had more options than its host. The virus could profit from the fact that, in its area of endemicity, the decrease of chimpanzees was paralleled by an handy increase of humans. Humans are physiologically close to chimpanzees and about equally susceptible to SIV, so adaptation was relatively easy.

This general scenario can be applied to HIV-2, although its host was not endangered. Sooty SIV continues to circulate in West African sootys, while HIV-2 circulates in West African humans. So why did it jump to humans from the abundant sootys? Because humans were there. From our point of view, we can see that in the long run, humans extend the range of sooty SIV because they are much more mobile than monkeys. But the virus cannot see that. In a sense, viruses are simply opportunistic, so SIV jumped to humans just because they were susceptible and available. Any virus, wherever it finds itself, simply tries to survive and spread. A sooty SIV woke up one day in the human bloodstream, perhaps after a monkey bite. It might have died in another host but was able to replicate to transmissible levels. The virus adapted to circulating at a low level and causing relatively little harm in humans (i.e., infecting and killing slowly) compared with other HIVs.

No matter how or why a virus changes hosts, we know it suddenly confronts a new set of cells to infect. These cells look somewhat familiar but are not perfectly accommodating. Perhaps the virus is drawn to the right cell receptor and can interact to infect the cell with modest efficiency but cannot reproduce too well. Gradually it adapts during the subsequent replication cycles. As already explained, the fittest viruses of the population—those that can best multiply to high levels—survive each cut and reproduce themselves, whereas less fit viruses disappear. What finally evolves is a population of viruses that replicate at a level that enables the virus to spread efficiently in the new host population.

This or any other adaptation (e.g., a recombination event to increase infectivity) may or may not cause detrimental health consequences in the host. For a virus, the meaning of life is survival and spread. It seeks only efficient reproduction and transmission in the host population at hand. Virus-host adaptation is a balance between virus virulence and host resistance. Both host and virus must survive long enough to produce offspring. However, the virus must survive only that long whereas, in general, the host must survive to produce and then raise the offspring.

Chapter 10 told how SRV thrived harmlessly in the wild, in a single species of African monkey, then became a monster that killed several species of Asian monkeys in primate research centers around the world. The story is yet another example of an AIDS epidemic caused by human behavior. For it to happen, humans had to remove the accustomed host of SRV from its natural surroundings and place it close to unaccustomed animals that were extremely sensitive to the virus: the Asian macaque. SRV did what came naturally, and not for the first time either.

Much earlier, this virus was born when an SRV ancestor found itself in an entirely new family of animals. As told in Chapter 10, SRV is actually a rodent retrovirus that acquired a monkey retrovirus envelope so it could spread efficiently in primates. Two endogenous retroviruses—a mouse virus and a monkey virus—were involved in this event. A mouse bite probably transferred a few mouse cells to a monkey. The contact of mouse and monkey cells could have activated an endogenous virus carried by the mouse cells. It shed virions that entered certain monkey cells. Meanwhile, the contact of mouse and monkey cells also activated an endogenous monkey virus. It shed virions that entered the same cell as the mouse virions. The two viruses mated, and the mouse virus ultimately picked up a monkey envelope. This enabled it to interact with a key molecule on the surface of a particular host cell.

A whole set of monkey viruses share an affinity for this same receptor. Some are exogenous like SRV. Some are endogenous like the colobine D-type virus CPC-1 and the C-type baboon virus BaEV. As explained later, it is important that BaEV only recently entered the germ line of baboons. This makes it an endogenous virus that can sometimes produce exogenous particles.

SRV shows how a mouse virus, needing to spread among monkeys, took advantage of viral sex to gain, by chance, a gene just for that purpose. The environmental pressure on the mouse virus in a monkey cell environment is its limited ability to enter and multiply in its new microenvironment, the monkey cell. The acquisition of a monkey envelope is all that it needs to become a monkey virus.

A virus has microscopic vision (though, of course, it cannot actually see), whereas humans have macroscopic vision. When we think of a monkey virus, we think of its host animal as a whole. When we talk about environment, we think of animal habitat. But for a virus, environment is the particular cells in which it can or cannot multiply. The monkey cell environment pressured the mouse virus to become a monkey virus by acquiring an envelope that allows attachment to a specific cell receptor. The cell receptor is the center of the universe for a virus: it permits cell entry, without which the virus cannot multiply. If it cannot multiply, it cannot survive in that particular environment.

The receptor used by SRV and other D-type monkey viruses is used exclusively by primate viruses with one exception: an endogenous virus of small cats. Known as RD-114, this retrovirus is found only in the domestic cat, the jungle cat, and the African wildcat, presumed ancestor of the domestic cat. The virus is totally absent from big cats like lions, leopards, tigers, jaguars, and cheetahs. Apparently it entered the germ line of cats after the evolutionary separation of big and small cats. It must have been acquired in the Mediterranean area from a local animal. This was probably the baboon, since BaEV is the nearest relative to RD-114. Cats could easily have gotten the virus from baboons when sharing the natural African habitat or the man-made Egyptian habitat.

Clues to the monkey virus parent of SRV may come from a close look at other D-type monkey viruses. Of the monkeys that carry those viruses, can we find one whose habitat overlaps with the talapoin? The African black colobus overlaps but is so scarce that it rarely meets talapoins. Baboons and Asian colobus are plentiful but do not overlap with talapoins. So there must be a missing link: a go-between animal that was infected by a virus of baboons or Asian colobines, then passed the virus (or at least its envelope) to talapoins. The evidence suggests the go-between was a mandrill, as will be explained.

The BaEV of baboons, a C-type virus, is usually endogenous and totally inert. However, being quite newly integrated into the baboon genome, it retains its own complete genome in at least some baboon cells. This complete genome can be activated to generate exogenous virus. Other monkeys carry BaEV, but only baboon BaEV can be activated. This is important to our story because, although sex and recombination are remotely possible when one or both partners are endogenous, the process is far more likely—and far less cumbersome—when at least one is exogenous. Ideally, a mouse virus picking up a monkey virus envelope needs both its parent viruses to be infectious particles when they meet.

Our work has demonstrated that in an individual baboon only a few (if any) cells carry complete BaEVs. But in a baboon that carries such BaEVs, activation by invasion of foreign cells can generate virions able to infect and reproduce. The process typifies the way an endogenous virus can become an exogenous virus in response to environmental pressure. The invader cells can come from other monkeys, from humans, even dogs and bats—or a mouse bite. In other words, baboon BaEV is xenotropic.

Most African monkeys have been thought to carry BaEV, but our work has not confirmed this (Figure 11.1a,b). When we checked our family tree of African monkeys for BaEV viruses that include envelope genes (the key for entrance to the monkey world), only a select group of monkeys qualified. Essentially, BaEV is present only in baboons and other Papionini monkeys and in the four subspecies of African green monkey. This shows remarkable coincidence with SIV, with two very important exceptions. Unlike SIV, BaEV is not found in chimpanzees and humans, nor is it found in guenons other than African green monkeys. Still, it seems clear that two monkey families—guenons and Papionini—govern most of the retrovirus evolution among primates, since they bring together endogenous viruses like BaEV and exogenous viruses like SRV, STLV, and SIV. To study virus adaptation to new primate environments, we have only to look at the habitat of these two families.

Habitat was obviously a factor in the spread of SIV between sabaeus monkeys and sooty mangabeys. Our work convincingly shows it was equally a factor in the distribution of BaEV. Whereas one group of mangabeys clus-

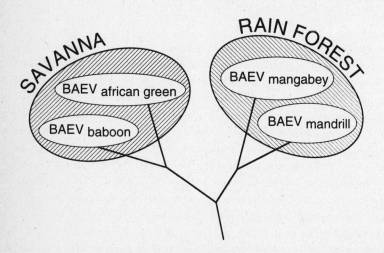

Figure 11.1a **Family tree of baboon endogenous virus.** *BaEV hosts are divided between forest monkeys and savanna monkeys.* (van der Kuyl, Dekker, and Goudsmit 1995b.)

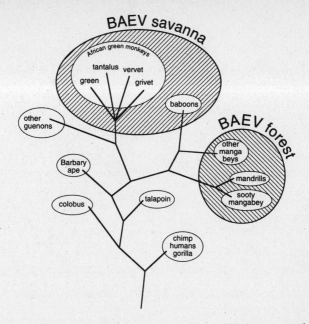

Figure 11.1b *BaEV infects African green monkeys and baboons, mandrills, and various mangabeys (but only in baboons can BaEV produce infectious particles). Many primates are not BaEV-infected, including the Barbary ape and great apes.* (van der Kuyl, Dekker, and Goudsmit 1995b.)

ters genetically with olive and chacma baboons and another group clusters with mandrills, the BaEVs of all mangabeys cluster with the BaEVs of mandrills. The BaEVs of baboons cluster with the BaEVs of African green monkeys, although the monkeys themselves are not genetically close. Clearly the virus clusters follow habitat more than species separation (Figure 11.2a,b).

BaEV seems to branch into forest viruses and savanna viruses (Figure 11.1b). The former have concentrated on forest primates like mangabeys and mandrills. The latter have focused on savanna primates like baboons and African green monkeys. Since the talapoin is a forest monkey, we must assume that SRV derived its primate envelope from an endogenous BaEV of some other forest monkey: a mandrill or a mangabey. One of these could well be our missing link between baboons and talapoins, and geography favors the mandrill.

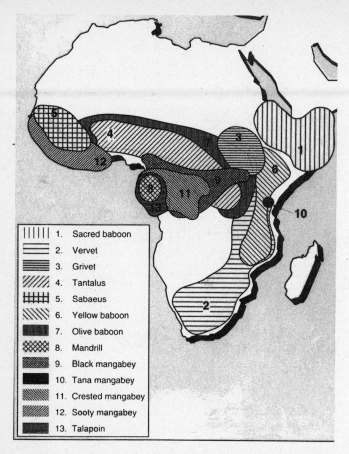

Figure 11.2a   Geographic distribution of BaEV. *Map locates all BaEV-infected African species of nonhuman primates.* (Ilynskii et al. 1991; van der Kuyl, Dekker, and Goudsmit 1995b.)

All known monkey viruses seem to predominate in one habitat or the other. Those that are strongest in the forest include some BaEVs plus SRV and SIV. Those strongest in the savanna include the other BaEVs plus STLV and the simian foamy viruses. All the BaEVs plus SRV and SIV seem restricted to African monkeys, but STLV and the foamy viruses—also called *spumaviruses*—infect monkeys around the world. STLV was long limited to Asia but finally landed in Africa and spread to the New World.

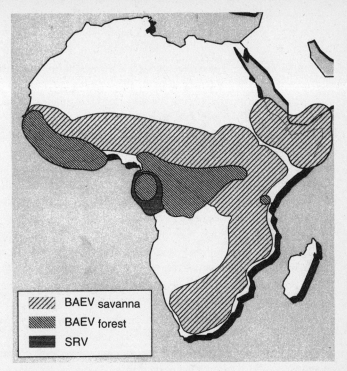

Figure 11.2b *Map shows BaEV distribution by savanna and forest; also SRV distribution in talapoin habitat.* (Ilynskii et al. 1991; van der Kuyl, Dekker, and Goudsmit 1995b.)

Simian foamy virus is even more widespread, infecting Asian, African, and New World monkeys and higher primates such as gorillas, chimpanzees, orangutans, and humans. It may be the most ancient of monkey viruses since it infects all its hosts without the slightest detrimental effect.

Simian foamy virus is the ultimate happy retrovirus. It never meets a primate it doesn't like. This retrovirus finds all primate hosts equally attractive and never encounters a primate environment that is hostile to its dissemination and spread. Its hosts are also happy (so far) because this virus does not need to adapt in ways that cause disease or death.

As we know, only a hostile environment forces the need for increased virus load for more efficient spread. When a monkey virus encounters a monkey of the preferred host species, no adaptation upon transmission is required since multiplication is optimal. But when a less preferred but susceptible host is encountered, virus multiplication is usually minimal at first. In the body of this new host, the virus will begin to evolve toward a new optimum, and the fittest (i.e., best-replicating) viruses will survive. These survivors will subsequently go on to the next host. HIV shows how this process can involve heightening the virus load, causing AIDS and the death of the host. BaEV and SRV show a different way to enhance virus spread. Instead of heightening the virus load like HIV, a virus can acquire a better envelope. This option was used in the case of cross-species transmission from mouse to monkey.

All of these observations indicate that the microenvironment of a virus—the preferred cell and its hospitality to virus entry and multiplication—is closely linked to the macroenvironment, the host that houses the preferred cell. In fact, the host provides more than housing. It serves the virus as a means of transport to the cell. From a retrovirus perspective, the host is a vast conglomerate of cells that exist only to support various activities that get the virus to its desired cell. These activities must enable the virus to pass from one individual to another, enter the body by a certain cell type, travel by a certain route to its target cell type (i.e., where it can multiply), then interact with the cell receptor to enter and cause infection.

Unfortunately for the virus, the host has an immune system to fight foreign intruders. When running smoothly, this system does not distinguish between good and bad but only between self and non-self. Otherwise it would damage the host, as it does in autoimmune disorders like rheumatoid arthritis. The system ignores all elements that are part of the host while attacking all foreign proteins. These include antigen, the protein (or perhaps several) unique to each invader that provokes the immune system to generate antibody specific to that invader.

Unfortunately for us, our immune system may be effective at the onset but finally is ineffective against HIV. Despite an immune response that includes antibodies and T cells to fight HIV, the HIV-infected individual almost invariably develops AIDS and dies from the inability to fight off normally innocent viruses, bacteria, and parasites. This inability is immunodeficiency or immunosuppression. In theory, disease should be prevented by HIV-specific immunity, which ideally should also clear HIV from the system. HIV simply does not provoke a very effective immune reaction in humans. In the laboratory, potent anti-HIV immunity has been found in the blood of infected individuals, yet almost never can such immunity prevent

AIDS once someone is HIV-infected. This suggests strongly that the virus is able at each phase of infection to reach new susceptible cells without much obstruction from anti-HIV immunity.

From the virus point of view, host immunity hampers adaptation to new host environments. The more effective host immunity, the more restricted the virus in seeking the best way to survive. In HIV infection, host immunity seems to be a small obstacle for the virus. The HIV virus loads generally remain extremely high throughout the course of infection, and only a tiny percentage of infected individuals escape immunosuppression and death.

Based on these observations, one can predict that in AIDS, the virus-host adaptation to an equilibrium happens fast, since virus and its desired cell meet virtually unimpeded. The absence of effective anti-HIV immunity makes it very easy for HIV particles to reach their goal because the road is unblocked, except by small speed bumps. All they need is the urge to arrive at the right cell, and this is driven by the chemical affinity of the viral envelope for a particular receptor.

Members of the HIV family share many features and strategies in addition to their affinity for meeting place. But viruses outside the family can also rendezvous (and ultimately mate) with HIV if only they share this affinity for the same cell type in the same type of host. This one common interest can bring potential partners to the same place, attracted by the cell receptor.

One can imagine that as any virus moves through a new host, it scans the total cell population and all the receptors offered to its envelope. It looks for the special cell type or types offering the molecule that fits the viral envelope. The molecule and its corresponding envelope protein are like a lock and key. Some keys fit only a single lock. Others fit multiple locks and, conversely, some locks respond to multiple keys. The first case represents the virus with high specificity for a given unique cell type. The second represents a virus able to enter a given cell in many ways through different receptors. The third case is analogous to cell types that can accommodate more than one type of virus.

As we watch for HIV to mate with another retrovirus, the third case is most important. Whether it invites multiple viruses by one or several receptors, this kind of cell provides a rendezvous for recombination.

However, it is easy to see that for the best chance of meeting, two retroviruses should share more than a taste for the same target cell. They should also share port of entry into the body. Once inside the body, viruses infect the first available cells of the right type. So if one virus enters through the mouth and the other through the anus, they are unlikely to come together. They will head for the same type of target cell but at opposite ends of the body. Viruses with different ports of entry rarely meet without development of generalized infection. This puts both viruses into the bloodstream.

As discussed earlier, HTLV-I and HIV-1 seldom meet because HTLV-I mainly infects children of breast-feeding age, by the oral route, whereas HIV mainly infects people of reproductive age, usually through the mucosal wall of the genital or anal tract. The danger is that HTLV-I infection can cause transformation, or unlimited growth, of CD4+ cells in the bloodstream. In this state the cells are highly vulnerable to HIV-1 infection, and thus to infection by HIV-1 along with HTLV-I. The dual infection can enhance the effect of either virus or both. It may lead to phenotypic mixing or, in the end, to the creation of hybrid or recombinant offspring.

Viruses spread opportunistically into any hosts that give them entry and allow them to replicate. Retroviruses continuously adapt to changes in their microenvironment. The most dramatic selective pressure for adaptation occurs when the virus finds itself in a new host, as when SIV cpz jumped to humans and became HIV-0 and HIV-1. It is in such instances that phenotypic mixing and viral recombination are most likely to occur. In the modern world of population and environmental change, retroviruses are ever more threatened with the loss of natural hosts and the need to find new hosts, including us.

There is perhaps some logic in our vulnerability to primate retroviruses since our activities are the major threat to rain forest animals not only in Africa but in all parts of the world. The most frequently mentioned habitat disturbance is logging. Common opinion is that, within twenty-five years, no undisturbed rain forest will be left. However, commercial logging is usually selective, taking not more than a tenth of the trees in a given area. So the issue is whether the loggers focus on trees vital to certain groups of monkeys, and whether these monkeys are vital to certain retroviruses.

Generally speaking, the larger-sized monkey species are more vulnerable to habitat disturbance than smaller species. In addition to body size, diet plays a role. If a monkey depends for its survival on fruits, it is more sensitive to habitat disturbance than a monkey that relies on leaves. Of course there are always exceptions. In Asia it turned out that fruit-eating macaques are very opportunistic and that some of them, like Indonesian macaques (*Macaca fascicularis*), are more common in disturbed forests than in undisturbed forests. Several macaques seem to prefer disturbed forest, resembling humans in this respect. In the case of *M. nemestrina* on Sumatra and *M. nigra* on Sulawesi, the preference is due in part to their habit of raiding crops, a habit they share with the African talapoin.

In Africa, the continent most important to our story, commercial logging dates from World War II, when African mahogany began to be logged for export. This logging was large-scale but quite selective. Meanwhile, logging for domestic trade was small-scale but less selective. It took important food trees, with effects that were especially hard on chimpanzees. Chimpanzees thrive poorly in disturbed forest because they rely on fruit (to a greater extent than the more versatile Asian macaques). Yet gorillas do well in heavily logged forests because they eat leaves.

African green monkeys adjust extremely well to habitat disturbance. Most guenons can make the best of a changed habitat because they are relatively small and not picky about diet or other living conditions. Striking differences, however, can be noted among guenons. The blue monkey (*Cercopithecus mitis*) is a generalist that can stand major habitat disturbances. Blue monkeys eat what they can get: fruits, insects, and leaves. In contrast, the redtail monkey (*C. ascanius*), which often breeds with the blue monkey in shared habitats, is extremely dependent on a single food source: the fig tree. One can imagine that this monkey has a hard time when fig trees are being cut down.

Colobines, like guenons, show a range of reaction to habitat disturbance. For example, *Colobus guereza* tolerates logged habitats despite meager food supplies, perhaps because it can tolerate a low-quality diet and needs to preserve energy by avoiding the cool temperatures of extreme shade. However, the African black colobus depends on the seeds of certain scarce trees to complete its poor leafy diet. The logging of these trees has very likely led to the endangerment of this neighbor of talapoins in the western equatorial rain forest.

Since habitat disturbance is not always harmful, one suspects it is not the most important environmental threat to nonhuman primates. Nor is it the greatest threat to the retroviruses that depend on these animals. Both the animals and their viruses are far more threatened by direct assaults: attacks on one primate by another. Human and nonhuman primates eat other primates. In addition, humans capture nonhuman primates for export around the world as pets, zoo animals, or laboratory models.

If we focus on the western equatorial rain forest, where many retro-viruses met their first human host, we find communities of talapoins, chim-panzees, mandrills, gorillas, and a few colobines, as well as humans. All are part of the ecosystem that modifies retrovirus host availability. As will be described, this ecosytem is nothing more than a food chain: humans eating humans (in the not-too-distant past), humans eating monkeys, monkeys eating other monkeys. Such a system offers ample opportunity for the cross-species transmission of viruses.

Africans of this rain forest area include the Fang or Fan, a tribe living in Mbini, the southern part of Cameroon, and the northern part of Gabon. The Fang were cannibals until the turn of the last century, according to Paul Belloni du Chaillu (see Chapter 5), who in 1861 published *Explorations and Adventures in Equatorial Africa*. He wrote that the Fang did not hunt people but purchased corpses. They used these for food, not ritual purposes. They habitually bought corpses from neighboring tribes, some-times trading them with other cannibal tribes like the Osheda. Apparently, all these cannibals had qualms about eating their own people. But some-times the Fang would buy corpses within their tribe, as long as they were outside their own family. When demand for meat was high, deceased slaves were purchased from the Mbicho and Mbondemo tribes at the price of one elephant tusk for a body.

Du Chaillu reports that the Fang cooked the body parts and sometimes smoked them before eating. Besides human meat, they lived on manioc, yams, squashes, and plantains. Their cannibalism is confirmed by Mary Kingley's *Travels in West Africa*, published in 1897. She was told by local sources that the Fang bought and sold human bodies as food. However, the Fang ended their cannibalism in the early 1900s, most likely because of pressure from the Spanish administrators of Mbini (then Río Muni) and the preaching of Spanish missionaries. Thereafter, like neighboring tribes, the Fang ate no higher primates than chimpanzees and gorillas.

Besides the Fang, few other tribes ate human meat, but monkey and ape meat were staples. In contrast to humans, which apparently were eaten only when they died of natural causes, monkeys and apes were actively hunted. Du Chaillu went on many ape and monkey hunts and tells of the killing of chimpanzees and gorillas by himself and local hunters. He de-scribes vividly how much these men liked gorilla meat. After a kill, they would quarrel over who got which part. When du Chaillu gave each man his share, it was eaten with great enthusiasm.

The practice of eating monkeys and apes, by the Fang and other people of the western equatorial rain forest, has declined but not disappeared. Fieldwork among the Fang in 1968 by Jorge Sabater Pi of the Zoological Gardens of Barcelona and Colin Groves of Cambridge University provided some crucial data. It confirmed that past or present hunting in that area could be a major factor in retroviral dissemination. Hunting contributes in two ways: by decimating natural hosts and by increasing monkey-to-human contact, making transmission not only inevitable but bound to happen more regularly.

According to one-third of the individuals questioned by Pi and Groves, the Fang prefer higher primates as food. The most favored are mandrills, although increasing scarcity makes these animals an infrequent meal. Guenon meat is eaten most often but is considered a staple, not a delicacy. The Fang avoid eating black colobus monkeys, which they consider dry and bitter, so at least for that species hunting is less a threat than habitat disturbance. Gorilla is now eaten rarely or only in secret, but older tribe members assured Pi and Groves that no meat surpasses gorilla meat. The most favored parts are the muscles, the palms and soles, and the tongue. During their fieldwork Pi and Groves were aware of at least five gorillas being killed for food. Interestingly, the Fang have no interest in chimpanzees. They disapprove of eating them, much as most Westerners disapprove of eating dogs. They eat chimpanzees only in extreme necessity. This distaste, if common in the region, perhaps adds evidence that humans did not get HIV from chimpanzees but from some shared prey like the colobus.

In the food chain, humans are a predator for gorillas, guenons, mandrills, and, to a lesser extent, for colobines and chimpanzees. This at least is true for the western equatorial rain forest, the birthplace of AIDS viruses like HIV-1 and HIV-0. Humans are not likely to reduce monkey and ape prey to zero because doing so would risk human starvation. But they may reduce these animals enough to interfere with spread of their retroviruses. Moreover, because of their predation, humans are routinely exposed to threatened retroviruses, which are bound to infect them.

Humans can be infected by eating a monkey, but infection is more likely to result from a monkey bite during a hunt. For two reasons this danger was greater in earlier times when hunting was done with bow and arrow. First, the hunter had to get closer to the animal to shoot. Second, a wounded animal was more likely to be alive and biting when approached for capture. With guns, the hunter can shoot from a greater distance and is more likely to make a deadly hit. The chance for prey to fight back is now dramatically reduced, but this only applies to hunting for food. Animals hunted for capture must be taken alive, so they can still bite their captors. When large monkeys or apes are taken, hunters commonly kill the mothers, but the babies can bite. Their panicked defense can cause injuries (and perhaps retroviral infection) but is less dangerous than the defense of adult animals. Young apes are not as large or as strong as adult apes, and they rarely carry the viruses that threaten us.

So guns have decreased the bites of monkeys hunted for food but have increased the bites of monkeys hunted for export. And habitat disturbance may make hunting easier for humans, further increasing their chance of being bitten. On balance, the risk to humans has probably risen. Theoretically, there is no reason why some still undiscovered primate virus might not eventually appear in humans. Depending on the level of adaptation needed to achieve efficient spread, such crossover could conceivably lead to new epidemics of fatal disease.

Of course, if predation or habitat disturbances drive monkey retroviruses to new hosts, these hosts may not be human but other monkeys. Habitat disturbance has many subtle and unexpected effects on neighboring animals of all kinds. A shrinking habitat may force two or more species of monkeys to live in a smaller area. This could cause them to fight more for food and territory, and perhaps to prey more on each other. For example, chimpanzees have long been predators of red colobus monkeys and several guenon species but have relied primarily on fruit. Disturbed habitats offering less fruit may cause them to eat more meat.

Clearly cross-species transmission of primate retroviruses could happen again, as when HIV-1 and HIV-0 entered the human population and SRV entered captive macaques. These transmission events represent only two of many possible scenarios. One involved local entry into the unaccustomed host population and subsequent dissemination over the globe. The other involved export of the natural host to a new environment occupied by unaccustomed hosts. Both cases plead strongly for stability in the natural host populations of primate retroviruses, to prevent future outbreaks of human disease.

Stability in these animal populations can only be achieved by leaving them intact. Whatever we think of "animal rights," for our own safety we must avoid human encroachment on these communities. We must also avoid the export of natural primate retrovirus hosts to unnatural environments where they can encounter susceptible species.

Individuals and social groups who are at low risk for diseases like AIDS must realize that the risks affect everyone. They affect people who never set foot in Africa or a gay bathhouse; never receive a blood transfusion; never see a prostitute, or engage in promiscuous sex. They threaten people who will never themselves be infected with HIV. When a retrovirus harms its host species, it harms not only the infected individuals but also the uninfected, mainly by curbing population growth. If too many disease victims die at or before reproductive age, their loss is also the loss of their potential offspring.

The direct and indirect damage caused by a retrovirus varies with certain factors, including the age and sex of those infected, the mode of transmission, and the level of disease fatality. An example of minimum damage is the epidemic of adult T-cell leukemia in southwestern Japan. The prime mode of transmission is by ingestion of breast milk, so individuals are infected before reproductive age. This by itself is threatening, especially since fertile women are affected. However, with HTLV, the threat is alleviated because although both men and women are infected, only women can transmit the disease. Men do not contribute to the spread of the virus, and unless women are unusually mobile, they infect only a few children. This keeps the infection very localized and, since few individuals actually develop adult T-cell leukemia, the death rate is very low. Taken together, these factors mean that the population effect of HTLV infection is virtually nil, despite a mode of transmission that allows for dramatic effects.

In contrast, HIV causes maximum damage. Being sexually transmitted, it obviously infects individuals at or before reproductive age. It infects both sexes and is transmitted by both sexes. Infected women can infect their offspring. If passed among strictly homosexual men, HIV-1B has minimal effect on population growth because these men are less likely to reproduce than heterosexual people. However, many homosexual men are actually bisexual. Also, particularly in certain cultures, heterosexual men have relations with women both vaginally and anally, partly for contraceptive reasons. So HIV-1B infects fertile women in Europe and the Americas. Other HIVs infect fertile women in Asia and Africa. Indeed, most Asian or African women infected by HIV are infected during their early years of sexual activity, their most fertile period. This is because HIV (mainly subtypes

1A and 1E) is endemic in the whole population, including sexually active males. Consequently, potential parents of either sex may die before they can reproduce or raise children. They may produce infected offspring who themselves will never live to reproduce.

Of course, HIV infection of fertile adults threatens more than population growth. It threatens not only the future but the present because a population ravaged by AIDS is increasingly a population of grandparents and grandchildren. The death of the people in between, the parent population, hurts not only the birth rate but the society in general. Many vital resources are eliminated because the parent population is also the population providing the resources. It is the men and women from puberty through middle age who most vigorously hunt, farm, and do most of the work that supports the economy and culture.

Survival of the uninfected population is therefore closely linked to the survival of the infected population. The larger the infected population and the higher the death rate, the more devastating is the effect on the whole retrovirus-susceptible group or species. So AIDS threatens all of us, directly or indirectly. And all of us must share the blame for this epidemic, regardless of our lifestyle or sexual orientation. The epidemic is rooted in human encroachment on primate habitats, and humans around the world began encroachment—on a large or small scale, by design or by accident, for profit or simply to eat—long before AIDS emerged in the last half of this century.

12

Human Survival:
Vaccines to Disarm HIV

Once upon a time, retroviruses invaded certain monkeys and apes of Africa. They came to these primates from rodents, cats, horses, or other ungulates, using viral sex to pick up fragments of envelope from primate viruses. These recombination events enabled them to enter and infect primate cells. In fact, their new envelope made them true monkey viruses, no longer able to infect their former hosts. Having jumped species, probably because of some environmental change, they could not go back because they had adapted too much. If some new conditions should force another jump, they might try the old host (if available), but the return would not be automatic. It would require adaptation all over again.

We have not yet seen a return or readaptation in the history of lentiviruses: no time when a virus moved to primates from another animal, then back again. The move from one host to another appears to be a one-way process if much adaptation is required. However, since viruses move by chance, they may jump just because a new host is handy. If little or no adaptation is necessary, viruses may not really leave the old host; they just add a new one and keep the old one too. This book has focused mainly on the viruses that move one way and leave forever their original host. But we have seen SIVs that have new and old primate hosts. We have also met a rodent virus (MMTV) that moved into primates (SRV and BaEV) and then into cats (RD-114), gaining new hosts and never losing an old one.

When a virus encounters a new host, it will remain if it can establish itself rapidly enough for transmission. Even if adaptation is long and difficult, the virus will remain as long as it can maintain at least some level of spread in the new population. If the host environment accommodates the newcomer well enough, an optimal equilibrium can be found between virus survival and host survival. This equilibrium may not be harmless to the host. If it is, it may not stay that way forever. But if we take SRV in talapoins, for example, and SIV in African greens or sooty mangabeys, for another example, we see that a virus with AIDS potential can be quite harmless to a host in which it has the chance to adapt optimally for its own survival. The issue of harm to the host will arise only when efficient spread requires destruction of cells crucial to host well-being and/or when it requires a virus load too high to be handled by host immunity. Apparently, neither is the case with SRV in talapoins or SIV in African green monkeys and sootys.

Since viruses are often assumed to become less virulent with time, some researchers believe that SRV and SIV were once harmful. They believe these viruses are attenuated, or weakened, in terms of disease-causing ability. This may be so, but we do not know and can never know for sure. We simply infer it from what we observe when SRV or SIV is transmitted to an unaccustomed host. When we see these viruses harm Asian monkeys, we assume they once harmed their natural African hosts. We see that several passages of SIV can increase virulence so that it infects more readily and kills faster. We may assume that continued passage would increase virulence to a point, then reverse the development, resulting eventually in an attenuated virus. But we cannot prove this. For example, to find out whether SIV might someday begin to lose strength in Asian monkeys—or whether they might become used to living with it—would require a prohibitive number of passages at a prohibitive cost of animal life and money.

What we can say for sure is that, whatever their virulence in the past, viruses like SRV and SIV can thrive generation after generation without doing harm to their accustomed host. We can also say that when SRV and SIV are faced with insufficient numbers of this host and simultaneously meet an abundant new host, they jump, spread, and cause the eventual death of individuals in the new host population. The fact that SIV or SRV in macaques can serve as a model for AIDS gives us some evidence that SRV or SIV cannot easily spread among Asian monkeys without harming them. But there are SIV strains that cause no harm to macaques whatsoever. We do not know their proportion in relation to harmful strains or how either kind would affect macaques in nature because neither would ever encounter macaques in nature.

Looking from monkeys to humans, we must note that while HIV tends to kill us, HIV-1 has no detrimental effect on about 1 percent of infected individuals. And HIV-2 has no detrimental effect on about 90 percent of the people it infects. HIV-2 spread in humans is minimal compared with the spread of the related SIV in sooty mangabeys and African green monkeys. Both viruses are relatively harmless in all their hosts. In contrast, HIV-1 spreads strongly in humans compared with the chimpanzee SIV. Though harmful to humans, it is harmless in chimpanzees in the wild.

So far we have no evidence from historical accounts that HIV-2 has ever been more harmful to humans—certainly never as harmful as HIV-1 is today. This suggests that from the virus point of view, the current level of HIV-2 spread is optimally adapted to the local West African environment. This is not to say that under different environmental conditions, such as HIV-2 now meets in India, the virus will not behave differently.

Since HIV-2 seems happy with circulation that is not widespread, we must rethink "widespread" from a virus point of view. To us, it has a global connotation, but to a virus, a small area may be wide enough. Currently, HIV-2 can sustain itself by infecting about 1 percent of West African humans, especially since SIV provides backup, continually crossing over from West African monkeys to start new strains of HIV-2. This SIV needs little help from its human variant to sustain the family. For generations it has infected 30 to 40 percent of adults among local African greens and sootys. Monkeys are its main reservoir, and what little is contributed by HIV-2 is incidental to family survival.

In contrast, humans are the main reservoir of HIV-1. Though the virus may have come to us from chimpanzees, it appears to be rare in those animals today. No other host for HIV-1 is known among primates or any other animals. The virus seems to rely for its survival completely on human dissemination, and humans have spread it beyond its original boundaries. Normally it would have remained limited to its original homeland in the western equatorial rain forest, but humans increasingly travel the world.

They now carry HIV (and all human pathogens) far and wide. The chances are close to zero that a human virus infection will remain confined to its natural ecological niche, as do the infections of most animals (unless those animals are transported by humans). So HIV-1 might have been happy with circulation in a very local human population, but we ourselves have carried it far beyond its natural evolutionary pathway.

Another way to contrast HIV-1 and HIV-2 is to look at their genetic closeness to related viruses. The SIV of sooty mangabeys is so closely re-lated to HIV-2 that some monkey strains are hard to tell apart from human strains. This means that SIV can shift to a human host as HIV-2 with very limited adaptation, perhaps none at all. The virus can just do its usual thing: when it finds itself in a human, it can replicate without much prob-lem. It reproduces a little less than in a sooty, perhaps, but can comfortably sustain itself.

One may say that this SIV is optimally adapted not merely to one species of monkey or primate but to a whole community of human and nonhuman primates. It is adapted to the shared habitat of humans and monkeys in West Africa. This must be paradise for a retrovirus. With a community of hosts, it has a foot in several camps and can afford to lose a host. If dependent on one host, the virus is always threatened with eviction and forced adaptation to a new environment. Multiple adaptations lead to virus flexibility in terms of hosts, which leads to virus survival at low cost to the population at hand.

BaEV appears to have made such adaptations. As described in Chapter 11, this virus separated in two major virus subgroups: $BaEV_{savanna}$ found in olive and chacma baboons and African green monkeys; and $BaEV_{forest}$ found in mandrills and mangabeys. In this instance, a shared habitat of-fered the virus the chance to spread in all the available and susceptible monkey populations. The virus-host equilibrium was reached when not one monkey species but as many as possible were infected. Apparently, the only limitation on the process was host availability, in other words, host habitat. The savanna and forest strains of BaEV must have branched apart before any monkey species were infected since we have found no common ancestor of the two BaEV families. Genetic analysis suggests that their separation must have occurred at least twenty-four thousand years ago. It must certainly have occurred before the Dahomey Gap was formed be-cause mangabeys and mandrills are both forest monkeys, yet they now live on opposite sides of the gap. However, individual monkeys sometimes cross over today, and perhaps have always been able to traverse this barrier. In any case, the BaEV story presents additional evidence that a retrovirus-host equilibrium may include multiple host species of the same susceptible host family. For a retrovirus, a community of hosts may be the highest state of being. The spread of SIV/HIV-2 as well as BaEV argues for this line of reasoning, though SRV offers an exception. SRV is apparently quite comfortable infecting only talapoins, even though humans are handy.

It has been noted that the virus load in SIV-infected but healthy sooty mangabeys is as high as the load of HIV-1 and HIV-2 in individuals who are developing AIDS (but much higher than in individuals not developing AIDS). Although this point is still debated in the scientific community, it appears to suggest that the level of circulating virus is indeed related to effective spread, but varies in its effect on the host species. Clearly, the sooty mangabey can remain healthy with an amount of virus in its body that makes humans very sick. This underscores the point made in Chapter 1 that progression to disease after HIV-1 or HIV-2 infection depends more on our genetic makeup (as a species and as individuals) than the makeup of the virus.

Obviously, we would greatly benefit if HIV-2 could outcompete HIV-1 in the human population, but this seems unlikely. No available evidence indicates that this is happening or will ever happen, at least in West Africa, where both circulate together. In that locale HIV-2 infects approximately 1 percent of the susceptible human population, and this rate has not risen over the last ten years. In contrast, HIV-1 subtype A is on the rise in West Africa and threatens to drive HIV-2 into oblivion in that part of the world. Despite its well-established monkey reservoir, HIV-2 could virtually disappear from humans in areas where HIV-1 has been introduced.

Studies conducted in Dakar, Senegal, by the Harvard group headed by Phyllis Kanki and Max Essex show that, under similar conditions, heterosexual spread of HIV-2 is much slower than HIV-1. Their data suggest that HIV-2 is less infectious and therefore less capable of maintaining itself than HIV-1 in a human population. Sexual transmission of HIV-2 is rare, and its perinatal transmission is even more rare compared with that of HIV-1. Since sexual and perinatal transmission are the most common routes in Africa, HIV-2 will lag far behind HIV-1 in a shared environment on that continent. Not only is HIV-2 slower to infect than HIV-1, but it is much slower to cause disease. In short, in a competitive situation, HIV-1 spreads well and usually makes the host sick. HIV-2 hardly spreads at all and causes disease, if ever, only several decades after infection.

An individual is undeniably better off with an HIV-2 infection than with an HIV-1 infection. In fact, in places like West Africa, where both viruses circulate, HIV-2 offers some protection against HIV-1. The Kanki and Essex group have shown that individuals infected with HIV-2 are less likely to be infected with HIV-1 than those who are not infected with HIV-2. They found that only after HIV-2 infection has caused a decline in CD4+ cells can HIV-1 infection get a foothold. However, this means that HIV-2 protection is only temporary and, once dual infection occurs, disease progression is faster than with either infection alone. Finally, we must remember that HIV-2 is an AIDS virus: it will ultimately cause AIDS and death when it manages to cause infection and disease. Its temporary protection against HIV-1 is nevertheless a good sign. It suggests that a weak AIDS virus has the potential to protect against a much stronger one, even when the two are as distantly related as HIV-2 and HIV-1.

Limited evidence pointing in the same direction comes from the rare individuals infected with HIV-1 who are long-term nonprogressors. These are individuals who escape impairment of the immune system for more than ten to fifteen years. Most of them can thank their own unusually good immune response and/or HIV target cells that are unusually poor at propagating the virus. But a tiny fraction of them (less than half a percent of all individuals infected with HIV-1) must thank their luck in catching an attenuated HIV-1 strain. For example, as recently reported by Learmont and Deacon, an Australian man is infected with an HIV-1 virus that lacks parts of certain genes and regulatory elements (e.g., nef and perhaps LTR) that are essential for efficient replication in the host. This man has shown no immunological disturbance by the virus after more than ten years of infection. When his infection was unsuspected, he gave blood to seven persons, who have been infected with his deficient virus. They also remain healthy to date.

This is good news, but with caveats. On the one hand, it is encouraging that such a weak virus is strong enough to infect target cells in the blood. On the other hand, both its presence in semen and its sexual transmissibility have yet to be determined. In addition, the lifestyle of all eight people puts them at low risk for AIDS, so their defective virus has not proven its strength against the highly aggressive HIV-1 strains that circulate among high-risk people. So we still do not know how well humans are protected by an attenuated HIV-1 strain. However, the Desrosiers group from the New England Primate Center has shown that macaques are protected against aggressive SIV by an SIV deficient in exactly the same way as the Australian HIV.

The big problem is that although attenuated HIVs may protect individuals, such strains are not likely to end the AIDS epidemic by outcompeting the more dangerous HIVs in the general population. This at least is true of the naturally attenuated strains we have seen so far. Whether HIV-1 or HIV-2, naturally attenuated strains simply do not spread efficiently. To do so, they would have to increase their production. This would probably make them more virulent, putting us back where we started.

Is there any way that a retrovirus can spread well while doing its host no damage? We all know the answer by now. It can, but only in the right host. African green monkeys and sootys, as well as talapoins, can cope with high levels of circulating virus without experiencing the slightest sign of harm from their SIV or SRV strains.

It seems likely, but cannot be proved, that when these populations were first exposed, most infected monkeys died. If so, a few males and females must have been able to survive infection. They produced offspring also able to survive infection, and eventually the monkey population—the ecological niche—was dominated by hosts that could coexist peacefully with the virus.

Another kind of coexistence has been seen among certain mice. The story starts early in this century when researchers developed AKR mice, a strain that is extraordinarily likely to get cancer of the thymus. When these mice are about ten months old, tumors appear because of a complicated series of events. First the mouse has an endogenous retrovirus that is activated soon after the animal is born. Early in the life of the mouse this endovirus produces circulating virions that are able to infect and reproduce. One of them enters a cell that harbors another type of retrovirus, still endogenous, which also sheds virions. The virions mate, and their recombinant offspring gains from the still-endogenous parent some gene fragments that allow it to enter cells of the mouse thymus. There it meets the virion of yet another retrovirus that is still endogenous. They mate and produce a recombinant with gene fragments that further add to its range of host cells. Once inside these added cells, it activates cell growth factors to facilitate its own reproduction. These cause the infected cells to proliferate like can-

cer cells, forming tumors. In the end, this cancer causes the death of virtually all affected mice about a year after birth.

Though discovered in laboratory mice, this intricate phenomenon also
occurs in a certain type of feral mouse. In this wild population it is offset by
another phenomenon: an intriguing case of retroviral protection against
retroviral disease. It was detected in studies by Murray Gardner, Christine
Kozak, and Stephen O'Brien of the University of California at Davis and
the National Institutes of Health at Bethesda and Frederick, Maryland.

In the late 1960s, Gardner captured many types of wild mice in southern California. Testing them for infection with cancer-causing retroviruses,
he found most types free of them, but one population was not. Gardner
had captured this population on a farm near Lake Casitas. Now called
Lake Casitas mice, they were found to be infected with murine leukemia
virus (MuLV). Over a period of observation, almost one-third of the animals developed disease: 18 percent had lymphoma and 12 percent had
paralysis of the hind limbs. Later two strains of MuLV were identified, one
causing the cancer and the other, paralysis. (See Figure 10.1 for the genealogy of MuLV.)

Since the infection rate was so high and about a third of the infections
were lethal, long-term survival of the Lake Casitas mouse population was
surprising. Even though MuLV-induced disease occurs only after sexual
maturity, the infection and its detrimental effects would be expected to
decimate these mice and eventually to wipe them out. This was especially
true since MuLV is primarily transmitted by milk ingestion.

So why did the mouse population and its virus continue to survive? It
turned out that a substantial proportion of Lake Casitas mice never became infected with MuLV despite its endemicity. This proportion was resistant even to direct injection of purified virus, whereas the rest of the
mice were vulnerable. A virus-host balance had somehow been established
in which the virus survived in the vulnerable population (which eventually
got sick and sometimes died), while the host population survived in its resistant members. If all Lake Casitas mice were vulnerable, they would
eventually die out, taking the virus with them, but virus and host had reached
a kind of détente.

During more than twenty years of observation, the Lake Casitas mouse
population was seen to remain MuLV-infected at a stable level of just over
50 percent. MuLV-induced disease remained the main cause of death
among these mice, but the virus did not overwhelm the population. Nor
did the number of MuLV-resistant mice grow to threaten virus survival.

This story shows that a retrovirus can sustain itself very effectively in a population that is partly susceptible to infection and partly resistant. In the vulnerable mice, the virus did not lose or gain virulence. Apparently, the 30 percent disease and death rate gave the virus enough susceptible hosts, particularly since the toll was taken after reproductive age. The virus could sustain itself because it was passaged to the next mouse generation during feeding of the newborns, before disease debilitated any infected mice. The Lake Casitas mouse population and its MuLV infection level remained stable because offspring of infected and uninfected mouse mothers were produced at about the same rate.

Gardner wondered exactly how the protective phenomenon worked. He found the answer by breeding AKR females with Lake Casitas males with and without MuLV infection. His question was, did mating with a MuLV-resistant male produce offspring resistant to the blood cancer or leukemia seen in all the AKR mothers? The answer was yes when the father was *completely* resistant, that is, he had two MuLV-resistance genes, one on both chromosomes. However, when the father was resistant but had only one MuLV-resistance gene, the offspring were split. Half were resistant and half were not.

What was this gene that protected some Lake Casitas mice against MuLV infection? As we know, a retrovirus enters a susceptible cell because the proteins on the viral envelope can attach to a receptor molecule on the cell surface. (As noted earlier, the envelope can be changed temporarily by phenotypic mixing and more permanently by recombination.) The moment cells are infected by a retrovirus, they become resistant to infection by retroviruses that use the same receptor. They are shielded by viral interference since their receptor molecules are saturated with bound envelope molecules.

In the MuLV-resistant Lake Casitas mice, the receptor molecules were found to be saturated. However, no sign of prior infection was seen. The mice were postulated to have an endogenous and crippled version of MuLV that expressed an MuLV envelope (or simply the envelope proteins) on the surface of susceptible cells. And indeed it was finally shown, by Hidetoshi Ikeda and Haruhiko Sugimura of the University of Tokyo as well as by the American group of Christine Kozak, that MuLV-resistant mice carry a truncated and noninfectious fragment of MuLV in all their cells (Figure 12.1). Because this fragment includes a viable envelope gene, an MuLV envelope was expressed to cover the cell receptors. If an infectious MuLV should enter the mouse and try to infect those cells, it found itself blocked. The

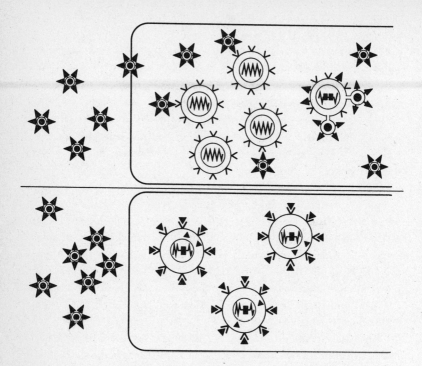

Figure 12.1 **Viral interference in Lake Casitas mice.** *Top left, exogenous MuLV invades a susceptible mouse. Its envelope proteins seek cell receptors, which are open to entry. At right, an MuLV-infected cell produces new virions (shown budding and cell-free), resulting in disease. At bottom left, exogenous MuLV is closed out. It cannot infect its target cells because every cell in the mouse contains endogenous MuLV. This produces envelope proteins that block cell receptors. Exogenous MuLV encounters viral interference as if infection had already occurred. It cannot infect a single cell in the body of these resistant mice. (Ikeda and Sugimura 1989; Kozak et al. 1984; Robinson et al. 1981.)*

deceptive envelope is like an "occupied" sign that warns visitors away from an empty hotel room.

One can imagine that the mice gained their resistance long ago when MuLV had become endemic and threatened the whole population. At some point, one or more ancestors were infected by MuLV as early embryos. When they were born, they carried bits and pieces of the virus in every body cell. MuLV had become endogenous to these animals. Probably in most cases, the fragments were a useless addition to their genetic material, but a few mice got a complete MuLV envelope gene. This made them resistant to infectious MuLV because of their endogenous capability to mimic viral interference. Over succeeding generations of mice, the resistant few grew into a substantial proportion of the population.

The bottom line is that, at this point, *all* Lake Casitas mice are infected with MuLV. About half have the exogenous virus that makes them sick; the others have the endogenous virus that keeps them well. Apparently, this situation benefits not only the mice but the virus; at least it does not threaten the virus. It shows that optimal host-virus interaction need not lead to the complete harmlessness of the virus in a given host population.

It seems to suggest a strategy against AIDS: the genetic engineering of humans to give them endogenous HIV that would express an envelope protein to fool exogenous HIV. Unfortunately, there are major problems with this model. First of all, HIV never infects the human embryo, so it could never become endogenous to humans. Even if it could, the treatment is too laborious (and AIDS already too widespread) to render all humans in the world resistant. If somehow this could be accomplished, we would not be resistant to all possible HIV strains but only to the most typical strains. Natural selection would then favor atypical strains that could threaten us in new ways. Needless to say, we cannot copy the Lake Casitas model by making only half the world resistant.

In California, most feral mice are not infected with either kind of MuLV, endogenous or exogenous. In both North and South America, most mice are descended from *Mus musculus domesticus*, a European mouse brought to the New World by explorers in the sixteenth century (Figure 12.2). None of the descendants of this mouse carry the retroviruses found in Lake Casitas mice.

One mouse that does carry these retroviruses is a Japanese mouse, *M.m. molossinus*. This rodent is a mixture of one Russian and one Chinese mouse strain. The former, *M.m. musculus*, came to Japan from northern Russia. The latter, *M.m. castaneus*, came from southern China. Both were no doubt brought to Japan when it increased trade with Russia and China in the seventeenth and eighteenth centuries. Based on features of the MuLV envelope genes (seen in various mouse subspecies) and our knowledge of mouse migration patterns, the Lake Casitas mouse is most likely a descendant of the Chinese mouse or one of its Asian variants. Unique among American mice, this rodent probably came on the ships that brought Chinese laborers to California in the nineteenth century.

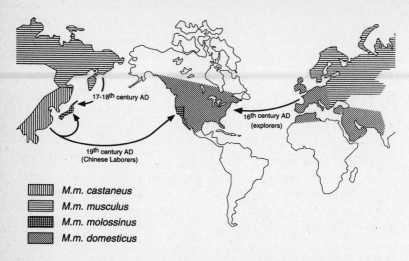

Figure 12.2 **US colonization by mice from Europe and Asia.** *In the six-teenth century,* Mus musculus domesticus *came on ships from Europe. This mouse dominates the United States except for a western pocket of* M.m. molossi-nus, *which came with Chinese laborers in the nineteenth century. Among American mice in the wild, only these are infected by MuLV, and about half are protected by endogenous MuLV. It is an unusual case of retroviral protection from retroviral disease.* (Gardner, Kozak, and O'Brien 1991.)

The second half of the last century witnessed an enormous exodus from China. Many Chinese traveled to places offering more opportunity than their increasingly crowded homeland. These travels were not without risk. They were often financed by the credit-ticket system, in which a voucher was paid on arrival by a relative, friend, or employer in America. When an employer paid, the immigrant repaid him in what was very close to slave labor. However, such an immigrant was considered free compared with the "coolies," contract laborers hired to work in foreign countries. Many coolies died on transport ships that were no better than African slave ships. But many survived, and, by the 1860s, two-thirds of the workers in the gold mines west of the Rocky Mountains were Chinese. The Chinese coolies and immigrants also worked for the big railroad companies, such as the Union Pacific and the Central Pacific. With them these Asians brought the ancestor of California's Lake Casitas mouse.

By now it is clear that retroviruses seek survival by achieving optimal spread in their host population. Among primate retroviruses, this goal is often reached through recombination. They took this path to become primate retroviruses in the first place. Then, having gained genes that code for a primate-specific envelope, they followed a number of very distinct routes to spread in certain primate populations.

Sometimes the route was short because optimal spread was readily achieved, as with SRV and the talapoins. Sometimes the route was long but relatively unpressured, as when the SIV of sabaeus monkeys moved slowly into the sooty population and gradually adapted to spread in both monkey species. Then, because of monkey-human contact, the sooty SIV became HIV-2. The SIV/HIV-2 family of viruses now circulates, relatively undisturbed, in two or three or maybe even more monkey species, as well as in humans. Whatever their host, members of this family have similar replication requirements, so they cause no disease in monkey hosts. In humans they cause disease of low frequency. Though very weak, HIV-2 provides protection against aggressive HIV-1 strains by some mechanism as yet unknown. Whatever the mechanism, we must remember that HIV-2 by itself may eventually lead to disease. And if HIV-2 infection is followed by HIV-1 infection, AIDS develops faster than with either virus alone. So HIV-2 is quite different from the innocent endogenous MuLV whose envelope gene provides protection with no strings attached.

HIV-1 is in a class by itself. The most dangerous of all AIDS viruses, it was pressured to jump from chimpanzees or colobus monkeys to humans. Its arduous route has involved splitting into subtypes, adapting, and spreading according to whatever conditions it met. By now, some subtypes appear optimally adapted to anal transmission, others to vaginal transmission. Either way, all HIV-1 subtypes eventually cause AIDS, and they do so more rapidly than HIV-2. HIV-1 appears to have no other major reservoir than humans, and, so far, its optimal spread could be achieved only with virus variants that are ultimately fatal.

No rapidly spreading and replicating HIV-1 strains have been identified that do not cause disease. This indicates that HIV-1 will not become harmless to its human host simply through natural selection for the best-spreading variant. On the other hand, HIV-1 continues to search for more efficient viral dissemination. It spawns more and more recombinants, particularly in Africa but also in Asia. HIV-1 subtype E, the virus that spreads most efficiently in Asia, is a stable envelope recombinant: a subtype A virus with a new coat. Subtype A appears to mate frequently with subtype C, another variant rapidly spreading in Asia. The virus seems to keep looking for the best configuration of its genes for optimal spread in the human population at hand, by the transmission route at hand. Its search may represent an opportunity for human survival. Perhaps one of its many recombination events will fortuitously yield a rapidly spreading HIV-1 that is harmless to us. Unfortunately, no evidence suggests that this lucky event is imminent, or even very likely. Somehow we must push HIV-1 evolution in the right direction.

Our best long-term strategy against AIDS is to develop a live vaccine. It must be an HIV-1 strain that is harmless (or relatively so) but spreads well enough in the human population to assure strain survival. It must also outcompete more harmful strains. It must be a strain that can take over and drive HIV-1 into oblivion, as HIV-1 now threatens to do with HIV-2 in West Africa. Such a strain is not likely to occur naturally. We have seen that naturally attenuated HIV strains do not spread well enough to outcompete dangerous strains. We must manipulate the development of the strain we need.

Meanwhile, in the short term, we must develop conventional vaccines that consist of HIV proteins, or antigens, that spark our immune system to defend us better. Science will continue to seek treatments that lower the level of virus. Ideally they will not only limit disease in the treated individual but limit viral potential to infect new hosts. However, we cannot be overoptimistic. Such therapies are on the horizon but will most likely involve drugs that will be far too difficult and costly to provide to the whole world, particularly to the people at highest risk: those living in poor areas without education or health services. Right now, brief treatment of pregnant women can often reduce perinatal HIV infection of newborns. It is not only costly but must be delivered just at the end of pregnancy. This narrow window makes it hard to provide even to affluent women, much less to poor women.

Increasingly, a constantly shifting combination of drugs is needed to keep up with shifts in HIV resistance. Even with the best combination, infections will keep spreading, and HIV may well develop multidrug resistance, making treatment harder and harder. Already drug-resistant mutants have begun to circulate that hamper the two-part goal of reducing disease and reducing infection of new hosts.

So how can we develop and distribute vaccines? The conventional type that elicits immunity may never completely prevent HIV infection. However, once infection occurs, such a vaccine could lower the circulating virus load, preventing spread of infection and progression to AIDS. This idea is feasible but, so far, no vaccines consisting of individually produced viral proteins have been tested in humans. Their development has been severely delayed by the lack of an HIV-1 animal model, a living humanlike system in which to observe vaccine effects.

Such an animal is still lacking, but we now have the next best thing. Classically, immunity to the all-important virus envelope leads to prevention of infection, or at least disease. Based on this concept, a virus was recently constructed, in the laboratories of Bill Narayan in Kansas City and Joe Sodroski with Norm Letvin in Boston, that wraps the genetic material of SIV in an HIV-1 envelope (Figure 12.3). Known as SHIV, it is SIV disguised as HIV-1. Passages in monkeys have shown these hybrid viruses to be able to replicate and cause disease. Produced by in vitro fertilization, they are man-made recombinants never found in nature. They have opened the way to test quickly all kinds of viral envelope vaccines for their efficacy in protecting against infection and disease development. The HIV-1 envelope of these hybrids will be recognized by T cells and antibodies that attach to its distinctive proteins. If a preparation of HIV-1 envelope proteins protects rhesus macaques against infection or disease caused by SHIV, the same preparation most likely will also protect humans against infection and disease caused by HIV-1.

We now have the means to find a safe and effective vaccine. We have the methods to monitor the shifting movements of HIV-1 strains. We know which viruses to watch and fear the most: HIV-1C and E in Asia and HIV-1A and C in Africa. But having a vaccine and knowing where to use it do not automatically get it to the people who need it the most. Distribution remains a frustrating problem. Regardless of where the AIDS epidemic started, the people now at highest risk are the most deprived in the world. They are concentrated in the poorest countries on earth, in the inner cities, among drug users, prostitutes, and neglected children. How can vaccines reach these people efficiently and consistently? Vaccines are less costly than therapies, but they can be nearly as hard to deliver.

A futuristic solution is to introduce HIV proteins in the food chain. The idea of edible vaccines was pioneered by Charles Arntzen of Cornell University in Ithaca, New York. Such vaccines would be simple and nonthreatening. Compliance would be assured since food is familiar, generally welcome, and often crucial for survival. The vaccines would be self-administered by those in need, not administered by outsiders often regarded with fear and suspicion.

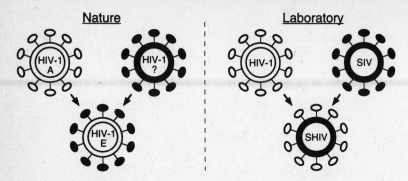

Figure 12.3   Viral sex in vitro produces SHIV to test HIV vaccines. *Born in the laboratory, this recombinant of SIV and HIV can infect rhesus macaques and make them sick. All its genes come from SIV except for an HIV-1 envelope gene. With its HIV-1 envelope, SHIV can serve as a challenge virus to test HIV-1 vaccines in rhesus monkeys, which normally resist HIV-1 infection. SHIV is reminiscent of what viral sex in nature produced in Thailand: HIV-1 subtype E. In that recombinant, all genes come from HIV-1A except for the envelope gene contributed by a mystery parent.*

In collaboration with Arntzen, we have succeeded in producing potatoes that contain HIV proteins. In fact, their genetic material has been augmented with genes that express HIV proteins (Figure 12.4). But this is only a start. Such proteins must be expressed at a higher level, and, instead of potatoes, they must be expressed in something like a banana: a food with broad climatic range that is natural to Africa, Asia, and South America; a food that can be eaten without cooking. Then, once the reengineered banana is eaten, the trick is to elicit immune response to the HIV proteins it smuggles into our system. Normally, foreign proteins are tolerated by the digestive tract so we can ingest and absorb nutrients. We would never survive if our immune system saw food as non-self and attacked everything we eat. So how can we get antibodies to attack the HIV proteins in bananas and not bananas as a whole or food in general? One strategy involves the genetic reengineering of the entire banana plant so that HIV proteins are not only expressed but encased in some kind of toxin. When the fruit is eaten, the digestive system will react to the toxin and trigger an immune response. The rest of the banana will be accepted as usual.

But if everything fails, we may still need a living vaccine, an HIV strain that will work for us. This evolutionary path might be our best long-term

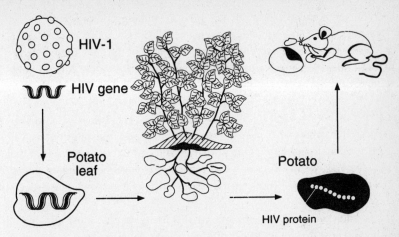

Figure 12.4 **Creation and use of an edible vaccine.** *The process starts with an HIV-1 virion, top left. The gene that codes for its envelope proteins is cloned from the viral genome and, by recombinant technology, is produced in potato leaves. The leaves are used to produce HIV protein in tubers, or the potatoes themselves. In the laboratory, a mouse that eats the potato benefits from heightened immunity against HIV-1. Such a vaccine in potato, tomato, banana, etc., could presumably immunize humans.* (de Jong et al. in press)

answer to AIDS. Viruses like HIV-1 do not care about spreading disease but only about spreading their genetic information. We can help them to our own benefit. For example, an HIV-2 strain might be genetically engineered to spread more vigorously while causing even less disease. Such a strain, if introduced into a population at risk for HIV-1 infection, might offer individuals protection against HIV-1 and, ideally, would outcompete HIV-1 in the population. But this kind of evolutionary project demands answers to many big questions.

First of all, it is not yet certain that the disease-causing effect of HIV-2 can be separated from its efficient spread and replicative capacity. The same is true for HIV-1 strains: all subtypes that spread efficiently appear also to cause disease. Second, though we have SHIV, we still lack an animal model for HIV-1 or HIV-2 as they appear in nature; this is because in nature no other primate or animal of any kind gets sick from HIV infection. Third and most frightening, only vigorous and well-replicating new HIV strains will protect against today's aggressive HIVs—but what if these new strains get out of hand? Can a vigorous and harmless virus be constructed without even the slightest chance of back mutation into a harmful virus? Desrosiers's macaque studies show that an SIV with a deficient gene causes no disease and offers some level of protection. But we do not know if such a virus might become harmful after several passages in the human population.

With its monkey reservoir, HIV-2 will pose some health risk to humans as long as humans and monkeys share the same ecological niche in West Africa. But protection against this virus is not our first priority since its threat is small and local. Our primary challenge is HIV-1. As with other types of HIV, we need a strain that replicates well in the genital or intestinal tract. It must protect against disease-causing viruses and cause no disease of its own.

In addition—and very important—this living vaccine must also spread from one host to another by sex or some other natural route. If a live, attenuated vaccine strain cannot spread naturally in the global community but can only replicate after injection in the body of a single host, its chances look poor from an evolutionary point of view. It probably cannot outcompete its naturally spreading and aggressive counterparts. And how can vaccine by injection reach all those millions in Asia and Africa who are currently at risk for HIV-1 infection? For every man, woman, or child injected with the harmless strain, many more individuals would be infected with the harmful strains. A concerted worldwide effort would be required to vaccinate every single person at risk for AIDS at such speed that the wild-type HIV-1 strains would suddenly find no unprotected humans to infect. The virus must be locked out so abruptly and securely that it has no time or place to adapt for survival.

Clearly, a big task lies ahead. We must know the AIDS virus very well to tame it, and already our knowledge gives us promising options. But we must recognize that science will find no quick or final solution to HIV or AIDS. Science alone cannot control this virus. Now that the HIV family has found the human family, it will always be with us in some form. All people must know HIV and work to control it. All people must know that HIV is only the first of a terrible series if we do not radically rethink our place—and our responsibility—in the world ecosystem.

Epilogue

The current worldwide AIDS epidemic is less than twenty years old, but its history is much older. AIDS is the unfortunate by-product of a virus's survival needs. We must remember that the underlying evolutionary requirement for survival of any virus is efficient spread. The evolutionary path in a new host population is therefore from slow and poor spread toward better and faster spread. Contrary to common assumptions, the path is not necessarily from more virulent to less virulent. Nor is it necessarily the other way around. As viruses improve their spread, virulence can change either way or not at all. What matters is the link between spread and virulence: the particular cell used—and sacrificed—for virus reproduction. If, as in AIDS, that cell is vital to host well-being, spread equals virulence.

The retrovirus that causes AIDS has come a long way from its original host. Even before it became HIV, it used sex—or, more precisely, recombination—to enter new host populations. It still uses this strategy to improve its infectivity and spread among humans, whatever environment or transmission route it encounters. Only when we recognize these facts and the nature of HIV can we conquer AIDS. We cannot stop this virus, but if we reroute its evolutionary path, we can hope to disarm it.

The three known AIDS viruses are all retroviruses of the lentivirus family, all descended from harmless SIVs. Two of them, HIV-0 and HIV-2, remain fairly confined to their original African ecological niches, most likely because they had little opportunity to move. In contrast, the virus that became HIV-1 jumped from its original host and found a foothold in humans. SIV cpz appears never to have achieved sufficient circulation in chimpanzees, which in any case became scarce. As HIV, it adapted rapidly and lethally to humans. In less than a century, the foothold has become a stranglehold.

At first the virus spread locally, in the western equatorial rain forest. Then, about the turn of the century, humans brought it out of the forest, probably to the German colony of Cameroon. From there some strains went to German East Africa, where the virus evolved into the African AIDS virus we see today. On the eve of World War II, other strains left Cameroon for Germany, where in some primordial form the virus began to cause AIDS. In Africa its virulence increased only when human-to-human sexual passage increased in the Lake Victoria area. Similarly, the virus became dangerously virulent in Europe only when its passage was markedly accelerated among highly sexually active gay men. In both instances, increased virulence was most likely a side effect of the increased virus load needed for efficient spread by vaginal and anal sexual routes.

Meanwhile, other retroviruses with similar cell tropism have been heading for a rendezvous with HIV and SIV. Again because of human interference, HIV and SIV now share various ecological niches with the human and simian tumor viruses HTLV and STLV. Viral sex has not yet been seen despite broad documentation of dual infections of STLV and SIV in monkeys and HTLV and HIV in humans. But the opportunity is there. Surely recombinant viruses with completely new properties will appear in time—perhaps a very short time—though recombination among these viruses appears to be less likely than it is among the various HIV-1 subtypes. The latter continually recombine as HIV-1 seeks to improve its survival in an ever-changing world. One recombination event has produced HIV-1 subtype E, which has already conquered Asia. This new strain appears to have gained efficiency in heterosexual transmission compared with HIV-1 subtype B, which spreads best by the anal route.

In addition to HIV and SIV, retroviruses like SRV have the capacity to cause AIDS and other life-threatening diseases but have yet to invade humans. SRV still circulates peacefully and exclusively among talapoins, African monkeys that are abundant and not at all endangered. SRV has not caused human infections in the talapoin habitat, although it is capable of infecting humans and talapoins regularly interact with humans. Stability of the retroviral environment appears to have kept such viruses in check.

Looking back, we can see that instability of the environment was a major factor in the rise of today's AIDS epidemic. Changes caused largely by humans occurred in the monkey and ape populations that originally sustained the SIV ancestor of HIV-1. Apparently the virus circulated almost exclusively among nonhuman primates. But as humans decimated these hosts they offered the virus an abundant alternative host. The virus made use of the opportunity and now depends on us for its survival.

Human interference continues and grows with the human population. Our intrusion on more and more monkey and ape habitats, especially the rain forest communities, has convinced some scientists that monkeys could vanish from the wild by the end of the twenty-first century. What will happen to their retroviruses? They will not simply vanish too. A few will survive in zoos with their remaining natural hosts. However, most of the monkey retroviruses will accept the opportunity to jump to new hosts, most probably to the human population. To survive and spread, they will adapt and cause disease.

One century is not much time to prevent these disasters, and already we have great damage to undo. One disaster can never be undone: HIV-1 is now among us and does its devastating job. Nonetheless, there are steps we can and must take as a unified global community. While scientists race to know and tame the AIDS virus, people everywhere in the world, rich and poor, must race toward two equally important goals. One is to protect the monkey and ape populations still extant in the wild. We must consider their survival needs along with our own and create more preserves and sanctuaries. The other goal is to protect human populations, particularly those of deprived areas and social strata, from the conditions that promote dissemination of HIV-1. This effort entails more and better education and health care: promoting safe sex, testing of blood supplies, using clean hospital equipment, preventing IV drug abuse and the use of dirty needles.

These goals may seem to ask an impossible level of collective and individual responsibility. One might question whether, even after education, enough people will be more careful of behaviors that can lead to HIV infection; whether they will be more caring about animal and habitat preservation. One can only answer that if we neglect these worldwide goals, the most sophisticated science, vaccines, and treatments will never tame HIV.

Glossary

accommodation A virus and host can reach a point of mutual accommodation, or equilibrium. Ideally, the virus can infect and spread comfortably, but the host suffers no ill effects.

anogenital Penile penetration of the anus. Anogenital sex is practiced most widely, but not exclusively, by homosexual men.

antibody An immunoglobulin molecule generated by the immune system in response to an antigen. It reacts specifically with the antigen and may remain indefinitely on call or can be rapidly recalled to react if that particular antigen reappears. The presence of antibodies therefore provides indirect but long-term evidence that infection has occurred, though some antibody is believed to occur naturally. (See **antigen**.)

antigen Any substance that, as a result of contact with appropriate cells, induces a state of sensitivity and/or immune responsiveness. This substance (e.g., a viral envelope protein) reacts with the antibodies and/or immune cells of the sensitized subject. *Note: Antigen* and *antibody* are defined in terms of each other. Like *deer*, both terms refer to one or many, but plurals are sometimes used, i.e., *antigens* and *antibodies*. Each antigen evokes at least one, often more, specific antibodies. (See **antibody**.)

asexual reproduction   Production of offspring that does not involve two parents and two sets of genes. The simplest organisms usually reproduce asexually by cloning themselves.

asymptomatic   Symptom-free; disease-free. An individual may be HIV-infected or HIV-positive but asymptomatic.

attenuated   An attenuated virus is one that has lost strength in its ability to infect, to cause disease, to reproduce, or to spread (any or all of these attributes). In this book the focus is on attenuation of disease-causing ability, or virulence. An attenuated HIV strain that infects, reproduces, and spreads is quite acceptable, if only it causes no disease.

bacterium   A one-cell microorganism that usually multiplies by cell division. Larger and self-sufficient, compared to a virus, it may or may not cause infection or disease.

BaEV/Baboon Endogenous Virus   An endogenous virus found in baboons and other African monkey species. In baboons, can become infectious; could have been a parent of the recombinant SRV of talapoins, the contributor of its primate envelope.

B cell   A B lymphocyte that resembles the bursa-derived lymphocyte of birds in its production of immunoglobulin. Unlike the T cell, it is short-lived and not directly involved in cell-mediated immunity. (See **lymphocyte, T cell**.)

CD4   A molecule on the surface of certain human T cells and macrophages, two types of immune cells. CD4 is a receptor or entry point for HIV, whose envelope proteins have an affinity for CD4 molecules.

CD4-positive (CD+) cells   Human T cells or macrophages that have CD4 molecules on their surface, making them susceptible to HIV infection.

clone (noun or verb)   Copy. The term refers to asexual reproduction and commonly implies *exact* copy. However, retrovirus clones are often inexact.

CMV/cytomegalovirus   A virus that often infects humans early in life. Usually harmless unless aquired too early or combined with HIV or other forms of immunosuppression.

colonization   Infection of one organism by another. May be short- or long-term; may or may not cause ill effects.

DNA/deoxyribonucleic acid   The nucleic acid that constitutes the primary genetic material of all plants and animals and some viruses. It duplicates itself and also acts as a template for synthesis of RNA, which produces proteins. Double-stranded DNA resembles a ladder wound into a helix, or coil. The ladder rungs are paired bases: adenine, guanine, cytosine, and thymine. The DNA helix is linear in chromosomes (mainly in the nucleus) but circular in mitochondria. (See **RNA**.)

endemic   An endemic infection has become natural to a population. Incidence and prevalence may be low, but the infection prevails and is almost impossible to eradicate. Like any infection, an endemic infection may or may not cause disease. If it does, virulence may be less than at the epidemic stage. (See **epidemic**.)

endogenous virus   A retrovirus native to an organism. It is heritable since all or part of its genome resides in the DNA of every body cell. Such a virus results when an exogenous virus infects an embryo before its cells differentiate. An endogenous virus is not infectious but, with a complete genome, may be activated to produce exogenous and infectous virions. (See **exogenous virus**.)

envelope, viral   Proteins that project from the virus coat (i.e., shell or capsid), forming a network of sites variously reactive to antibody, receptors, and so on. Each virus strain has certain distinctive proteins (see V3 signature site) but also shares many with related strains.

enzyme   Any of a vast class of proteins that perform various conversion and digestion activities in all living things. Their names typically end in *-ase*, e.g., reverse transcriptase.

epidemic (noun or adjective)   Refers to the occurrence in a community or region of more than normal cases of infection, disease, or other problem. It began as a human term but is increasingly applied to any group of organisms. An epidemic infection may or may not cause disease. It can run its course and disappear, or become endemic. (See **endemic, sporadic**.)

equilibrium   Mutual accommodation of a virus and host.

eukaryote   An organism distinguished from a simpler type by various features, notably a membrane-bound nucleus that contains the genetic material. (See **prokaryote**.)

exogenous virus   An infectious particle, i.e., a virus or virion able to enter and infect a new cell. Compare with **endogenous virus**, which is not infectious but can sometimes produce infectious particles.

family tree   The relationship of viruses, monkeys, or other organisms based on analysis of their genomes, genes, or gene fragments.

gay   See **homosexual**.

generalized infection   Not localized to one organ or system; has entered the bloodstream.

genetic analysis   Comparison of two or more cells or organisms based on differing nucleotides in a shared gene or gene fragment. Can establish history, relatedness, and grouping of types, subtypes, strains, and so on.

genome   The complete gene set of an organism. In eukaryotes this genetic material is packaged in a number of chromosomes; in prokaryotes, a single chromosome. In viruses, it is single or double stranded DNA or RNA molecules.

herpesvirus   A virus family including the recently identified agent of Kaposi's sarcoma. This agent is not of the herpes group linked to genital herpes, chicken pox, or shingles but is close to the Epstein-Barr virus, agent of mononucleosis and associated with certain blood cancers. (See **Kaposi's sarcoma**.)

heterosexual   In reference to sexual relations, lifestyle, HIV transmission, and so on, this term implies male-female pairing, or penile contact with the vagina. However, male-female couples may also have penile-anal contact.

heterozygous virus   A virus having two RNA strands, one inherited intact from the father and one intact from the mother. (See **homozygous viruses**.)

HIV/human immunodeficiency virus   By analogy, SIV, FIV, and BIV are simian, feline, and bovine immunodeficiency viruses but they rarely, if ever, cause immunodeficiency in their natural hosts. HIV types include HIV-0, HIV-1, and HIV-2; each is divided into various subtypes and, further, into many strains and substrains.

homosexual   In reference to sexual relations, lifestyle, HIV transmission, and so on, this term implies male-male pairing and anogenital intercourse, though not all homosexual men practice such intercourse.

homozygous virus   A virus having two identical RNA strands that mix the genetic material of both parents. (See **heterozygous virus**.)

HTLV-I and II/human T-cell lymphoma and leukemia viruses   Also known as lymphotropic viruses, these retroviruses are not lentiviruses but oncoviruses. They seldom cause disease or meet HIV in the same cell but are prospective HIV partners for production of recombinants. In monkeys they are STLV-I and II.

immune cells   Cells that participate in the immune defense system, for example, B cells and T cells (lymphocytes) and macrophages. The crucial T cells with a CD4 molecule on their surface are the main target of HIV infection. (See **lymphocyte, B cell, T cell, macrophage**.)

immunodeficiency   A condition resulting from a defective immune mechanism. It may be *primary* (a defect in the immune mechanism itself) or *secondary* (caused by another disease process); *specific* (a defect in the B-lymphocyte and/or T-lymphocyte system) or *nonspecific* (a defect in part of the nonspecific immune mechanism).

incidence   The number of specified new events (e.g., infections) in a population within a given period. Not to be confused with **prevalence**, the number or proportion of a population affected at one point in time. **Incidence** is most often used in this book.

infection   Colonization of one organism by another. The word commonly implies ill effects, but strictly it means only colonization. May be short- or long-term, harmful or harmless.

infection, acute   A short-term or brief infection; not **chronic** (repeated at intervals or lasting a long time). When applied to a harmful infection, acute often implies "severe."

infectious agent   A bacterium, virus, or other agent that can infect or colonize a host. An infectious agent causes infection but not necessarily disease.

infectious particle   An individual virus or virion. It is complete and viable, that is, it can infect a cell and reproduce. Incomplete particles can do only one or the other, or neither.

Kaposi's sarcoma (KS)   The tumor most often seen with infection by HIV-1B. It is otherwise rare in Europe and the Americas but quite common in Africa. Even in Africa, it is rarely serious unless combined with HIV infection. Characterized by bluish red skin lesions that start on the lower legs and move upward on the body; sometimes they move inward to organs such as lymph nodes. Putative agent recently identified as a herpesvirus.

Koch's postulates   Stated by German bacteriologist and Nobelist Robert Koch, the four kinds of evidence required to link a disease with its pathogenic agent: (1) the suspect organism must be found in every case of the disease in question; (2) it must be isolated and grown in culture; (3) when injected into susceptible subjects, it must cause the disease; (4) it must be observed in/recovered from each diseased subject.

lentivirus   Lentivirinae, a subfamily of "slow" viruses (family Retroviridae) includes HIV, SIV, and certain retroviruses of cattle and other animals.

leukocyte   Any white blood cell, of which about one-quarter are lymphocytes.

lymphocyte   An immunologically important white blood cell or leukocyte that is formed in lymphatic tissue. (See **B cell, T cell**.)

macrophage   These immune cells are called "big eater" in Greek because they destroy invaders by engulfing and digesting them.

MuLV/murine leukemia virus   A virus found in America among AKR mice in the laboratory and Lake Casitas mice in the wild. Unlike most American mice, the latter came from Asia, not Europe. About half of them have endogenous MuLV, which protects them against exogenous MuLV an example of retroviral protection against retroviral disease.

nonhuman primates   All apes and monkeys. (See **primates**.)

opportunistic agent   An organism that normally causes no disease but which, under certain circumstances, can cause opportunistic infection, such as *P. carinii*.

orofecal   Refers to oral or lingual contact with fecal material, perhaps incidental to oral-anal contact.

passage   The cycle that takes a virus from one host to the next, for example, SIV markedly increased in virulence after six passages in monkeys. Can be a verb, for example, SIV was passaged (cycled) six times through monkeys.

P. carinii   Abbreviation for *Pneumocystis carinii*, a widespread and opportunistic microorganism, probably a kind of yeast. It often infects or colonizes humans, usually without harm. However, when given the opportunity by HIV infection, it can cause fatal *Pneumocystis carinii* pneumonia (*P. carinii* pneumonia or PCP).

pneumocystis pneumonia (PCP)   See **P. carinii**.

primates   Members of the phylum Primata, considered the "primary," or most highly evolved, mammals. The name is commonly applied only to apes and monkeys, but humans are also primates. Apes and monkeys are properly called *nonhuman primates*.

prokaryote   A usually one-celled organism that is distinguished from higher organisms by its lack of true nucleus or chromosomes. (See **eukaryote**.)

recombination   A process by which genes or gene parts are exchanged to produce a recombinant, that is, a cell or an individual with a new combination of genes not found together in either parent.

retroviral sex   A two-stage process resulting in virus offspring having two identical RNA strands that are different from each parent, being a new mixture of both. (See **homozygous virus**.)

retrovirus An RNA virus with an enzyme that converts RNA to DNA so it can enter the host genome. This enzyme, reverse transcriptase, makes the retrovirus different from other RNA viruses and accounts for its name: "backward virus." Until its discovery, DNA conversion to RNA was well known, but never the reverse. Retroviruses were characterized by Howard Temin and David Baltimore, who worked independently and shared the 1975 Nobel Prize for medicine and physiology with Renato Dulbecco.

reverse transcriptase An enzyme, found only in retroviruses, that converts their RNA to DNA, so the viral genome can enter the host genome. (See **retrovirus, DNA, RNA**.)

RNA/ribonucleic acid The nucleic acid that forms the genetic material of RNA viruses and retroviruses. In retroviruses like HIV, reverse transcriptase converts single-stranded RNA to double-stranded DNA so it can enter the host genome. RNA has four bases: like DNA it has adenine, cytosine, guanine; unlike DNA, it has uracil, not thymine. Note: In organisms having DNA as genetic material, RNA is synthesized to make proteins. (See **DNA**.)

sequence Any series, but especially a stretch of nucleic acids (nucleotides) in genetic material; or a stretch of amino acids in a protein. To sequence (verb) is to determine the exact order of nucleotides or amino acids.

seroconversion The point at which signs of infection first appear/are detected. Signs include the presence of the infectious agent, its genetic material, antigen, or antibody. (See **seropositivity**.)

seropositivity The presence of signs of infection, for example, antibodies against an infectious agent. This is an ongoing state, in contrast to **seroconversion**, a point in time.

signature site A stretch of amino acids within a protein (or a stretch of nucleotides within a gene) that are unique to a virus or group of viruses, and thus serve as an identification marker. HIVs are identified by the **V3 signature site**, a sequence found in the third variable domain of an HIV envelope protein (or in the gene that codes for that protein).

slim disease Common name in parts of Africa for the wasting form of AIDS caused mainly by HIV-1A.

sporadic A sporadic disease is scattered, not epidemic. It may or may not proceed to the epidemic stage. (See **epidemic, endemic**.)

SRV/simian retrovirus A harmless virus of talapoins that has caused disease in Asian macaques. A rodent virus that gained a monkey virus envelope.

syncytia   Large, multinucleated cell clusters. In about 50 percent of HIV-1-infected patients, the virus changes as much as one or two years before AIDS develops and begins to cause syncytia in culture. The virus is then more transmissible to cell lines but probably less transmissible among people.

T cell   A T lymphocyte that originates in the thymus. A type of leukocyte or white blood cell, it is long-lived and responsible for cell-mediated immunity. Various types include helper and killer cells. (See **B cell, lymphocyte, leukocyte**.)

V3 signature site   See **signature site**.

virion   An infectious virus particle.

virulence   Damage or potential for damage. The more virulent a virus, the more likely and quickly it is to cause death of the host.

virus   An infectious agent that may or may not cause disease. Most viruses are smaller than the smallest bacterium and cannot be seen under the light microscope. Unlike bacteria, viruses lack independent metabolic functions and cannot grow or reproduce apart from a host cell.

virus load   The amount of virus, virus-infected cells, or virus-producing cells circulating in an individual.

wasting   Severe or persistent weight loss and emaciation that are not primarily caused by insufficient diet. An individual with a wasting disease can literally waste away.

Bibliography

Armitage, P.L., and Clutton-Brock, J. "A Radiological and Histological Investigation into the Mummification of Cats from Ancient Egypt." *J Arch Science* 8: 185–196, 1981.

Asher, D.M., Goudsmit, J., Pomeroy, K.L., Garruto, R.M., Bakker, M., Ono, S.G., Elliott, N., Harris, K., Askins, H., Eldadah, Z., Goldstein, A.D., and Gajdusek, D.C. "Antibodies to HTLV-1 in Populations of the Southwestern Pacific." *J Med Virol* 26: 339–351, 1988.

Åsjö, B., Albert, J., Karlsson, A., Morfeld-Manson, K., Biberfield, G., Lidman, K., and Fenyö, E.M. "Replicative Capacity of Human Immunodeficiency Virus from Patients with Varying Severity of HIV Infection." *Lancet* 2: 660–662, 1986.

Bada, J.L., Wang, X.S., Poinar, H.N., Pääbo, S., and Poinar, G.O. "Amino Acid Racemization in Amber-Entombed Insects: Implications for DNA Preservation." *Geochimica et Cosmochimica Acta* 58: 3131–3135, 1994.

Barré-Sinoussi, F., Chermann, J.C., Rey, F., Nugeyre, M.T., Chamaret, S., Gruest, J., Dauguet, C., Axler-Blin, C., Brun-Vézinet, F., Rouzioux, C., Rozenbaum, W., and Montagnier, L. "Isolation of a T-lymphotropic Retrovirus from a Patient at Risk for Acquired Immune Deficiency Syndrome (AIDS)." *Science* 220: 868–871, 1983.

Benveniste, R.E. "The Contributions of Retroviruses to the Study of Mammalian Evolution." In *Molecular Evolutionary Genetics*, ed. R.J. MacIntyre. New York: Plenum Press, 1985.

Benveniste, R.E., and Todaro, G.J. "Evolution of Primate Oncornaviruses: An Endogenous Virus from Langurs (*Presbytis spp.*) with Related Virogene Sequences in Other Old World Monkeys." *Proc Natl Acad Sci USA* 74: 4557–4561, 1977.

van den Berg, H., Gerritsen, E.J.A., van Tol, M.J.D., Dooren, L.J., and Vossen, J.M. "Ten Years after Acquiring an HIV-1 Infection: A Study in a Cohort of Eleven Neonates Infected by Aliquots from a Single Plasma Donation." *Acta Paediatr* 83: 173–178, 1994.

Bieniasz, P.D., Rethwilm, A., Pitman, R., Daniel, M.D., Chrystie, I., and McClure, M.O. "A Comparative Study of Higher Primate Foamy Viruses, Including a New Virus from a Gorilla." *Virology* 207: 217–228, 1995.

Boesch, C., and Boesch, H. "Hunting Behavior of Wild Chimpanzees in the Taï National Park." *Am J Phys Anth* 78: 547–573, 1989.

Bohannon, R.C., Donehower, L.A., and Ford, R.J. "Isolation of a Type D Retrovirus from B-cell Lymphomas of a Patient with AIDS." *J Virol* 65: 5663–5672, 1991.

Boxer, C.R. "List of Goods Imported by the Dutch to Japan in 1672–1674." *Transactions of the Asiatic Society of Japan* 7: 184–195, 1930.

Brown, E.W., Yuhki, N., Packer, C., and O'Brien, S.J. "A Lion Lentivirus Related to Feline Immunodeficiency Virus: Epidemiologic and Phylogenetic Aspects." *J Virol* 68: 5953–5968, 1994.

Busse, C.D. "Chimpanzee Predation as a Possible Factor in the Evolution of Red Colobus Monkey Social Organization." *Evolution* 31: 907–911, 1977.

Bygbjerg, I.C. "AIDS in a Danish Surgeon (Zaire, 1976)." *Lancet* 1 (8330): 925, 1983.

Chadwick, B.J., Coelen, R.J., Sammels, L.M., Kertayadnya, G., and Wilcox, G.E. "Genomic Sequence Analysis Identifies Jembrana Disease Virus as a New Bovine Lentivirus". *J Gen Virol* 76: 189–192, 1995.

du Chaillu, P.B. *Explorations and Adventures in Equatorial Africa*. London: John Murray, 1861.

Chen, J.L., Zekeng, L., Yamashita, M., Takehisa, J., Miura, T., Ido, E., Mboudjeka, I., Tsague, J., Hayami, M., and Kaptue, L. "HTLV Type I Isolated form a Pygmy in Cameroon Is Related to but Distinct from the Known Central African Type." *AIDS Res Hum Retroviruses* 11: 1529–1531, 1995.

Chen, Z.W., Telfer, P., Reed, P., Zhang, L.Q., Gettie, A., Ho, D.D., Marx, P.A. "Isolation and Characterization of the First Simian Immunodeficiency Virus from a Feral Sooty Mangabey (*Cercocebus atys*) in West Africa." *J Med Primatol* 24: 108–115, 1995.

Chopra, H.C., and Mason, M.M. "A New Virus in a Spontaneous Mammary Tumor of a Rhesus Monkey." *Cancer Res* 30: 2081–2086, 1970.

Clavel, F., Brun-Vézinet, F., Guétard, D., Chamaret, S., Laurent, A., Rouzioux, C., Rey, M., Katlama, C., Rey, F., Champelinaud, J.L., Nina, J.S., Mansinho, K., Santos-Ferreira, M., Klatzmann, D., and Montagnier, L. "LAV type II: Un second rétrovirus associé au SIDA en Afrique de l'Ouest." *C R Acad Sci Paris*

302: 485–488, 1986.

Coffin, J.M. "Structure and Classification of Retroviruses." In *The Retroviridae*, ed. J.A. Levy. New York: Plenum Press, 1992.

———. Reverse Transcription and Evolution. In *Reverse Transcriptase*, ed. A.M. Skalka and S.P. Goff. New York: Cold Spring Harbor Laboratory Press, 1993.

Cohen, J. "Can One Type of HIV Protect Against Another Type?" *Science* 268: 1566, 1995.

Corbitt, G., Bailey, A.S., and Williams, G. "HIV Infection in Manchester, 1959." *Lancet* 336: 51, 1990.

Cornelissen, M., Kampinga, G., Zorgdrager, F., Goudsmit, J., and the UNAIDS Network for HIV Isolation and Characterization. "Human Immunodeficiency Virus Type 1 Subtypes Defined by *env* Show High Frequency of Recombinant *gag* Genes. *J Virol*, in press.

Cornelissen, M., Kuiken, C., Zorgdrager, F., Hartman, S., and Goudsmit, J. "Gross Defects in the *vpr* and *vpu* Genes of HIV-1 Cannot Explain the Differences in RNA Copy Number between Long-term Asymptomatics and Progressors. *AIDS Res Human Retrov*, in press.

Daniel, M.D., Letvin, N.L., Sehgal, P.K., Schmidt, D.K., Silva, D.P., Solomon, K.R., Hodi, F.S., Jr., Ringler, D.J., Hunt, R.D., King, N.W., and Desrosiers, R.C. "Prevalence of Antibodies to 3 Retroviruses in a Captive Colony of Macaque Monkeys." *Int J Cancer* 41: 601–608, 1988.

Deacon, N.J., Tsykin, A., Solomon, A., Smith, K., Ludford-Menting, M., Hooker, D.J., McPhee, D.A., Greenway, A.L., Ellet, A., Chatfield, C., Lawson, V.A., Crowe, S., Maerz, A., Sonza, S., Learmont, J., Sullivan, J.S., Cunningham, A., Dwyer, D., Dowton, D., and Mills, J. "Genomic Structure of an Attenuated Quasi Species of HIV-1 from a Blood Transfusion Donor and Recipients." *Science* 270: 988–991, 1995.

Delwart, E.L., Sheppard, H.W., Walker, B.D., Goudsmit, J., and Mullins, J.I. "Human Immunodeficiency Virus Type 1 Evolution in vivo Tracked by DNA Heteroduplex Mobility Assays." *J Virol* 68: 6672–6683, 1994.

Diamond, J. *The Rise and Fall of the Third Chimpanzee*. London: Vintage, 1992.

Dietrich, U., Grez, M., Von Briesen, H., Panhans, B., Geissendorfer, M., Kuhnel, H., Maniar, J., Mahambre, G., Becker, W.B., Bechler, M.L.B., and Rübsamen-Waigmann, H. "HIV-1 Strains from India Are Highly Divergent from Prototypic African and US/European Strains, but Are Linked to a South African Isolate." *AIDS* 7: 23–27, 1993.

Downing, R.G., Eglin, R.P., and Bayley, A.C. "African Kaposi's Sarcoma and AIDS." *Lancet* 1 (8375): 478–480, 1984.

von der Driesch, A. "Affenhaltung und Affenverehrung in der Spätzeit des Alten Ägypten." *Tierärztl Prax* 21: 95–101, 1993.

von der Driesch, A., and Boessneck, J. "Krankhaft veränderte Skelettreste von Pavianen aus altägyptischer Zeit." *Tierärztl Prax* 13: 367–372, 1985.

Eigen, M., and Nieselt-Struwe, K. "How Old Is the Immunodeficiency Virus?" *AIDS* 4 (suppl. 1): S85-S93, 1990.

Elder, J.H., Lerner, D.L., Hasselkus-Light, C.S., Fontenot, D.J., Hunter, E., Luciw, P.A., Montelaro, R.C., and Phillips, T.R. "Distinct Subsets of Retroviruses Encode dUTPase." *J. Virol* 66: 1791–1794, 1992.

Emery, W.B. "Preliminary Report on the Excavations at North Saqqara, 1968–9." *Journal of Egyptian Archaeology* 56: 5–11, 1970.

Epstein, L.G., Berman, C.Z., Sharer, L.R., Khademi, M., and Desposito, F. "Unilateral Calcification and Contrast Enhancement of the Basal Ganglia in a Child with AIDS Encephalopathy." *Am J of Neuroradiology* 8: 163–165, 1987.

Essex, M., McLane, M.F., Lee, T.H., Falk, L., Howe, C.W.S., Mullins, J.I., Cabradilla, C., and Francis, D.P. "Antibodies to Cell Membrane Antigens Associated with Human T-cell Leukemia Virus in Patients with AIDS." *Science* 220: 859–862, 1983.

Estaquier, J., Peeters, M., Bedjabaga, L., Honoré, C., Bussi, P., Dixson, A., and Delaporte, E. "Prevalence and Transmission of Simian Immunodeficiency Virus and Simian T-cell Leukemia Virus in a Semi-Free-Range Breeding Colony of Mandrills in Gabon." *AIDS* 5: 1385–1386, 1991.

Fa, J.E., ed. *The Barbary Macaque: A Case Study in Conservation.* New York: Plenum Press, 1984.

Fenyö, E.M. "Antigenic Variation of Primate Lentiviruses in Humans and Experimentally Infected Macaques." *Immunol Rev* 140: 131–146, 1994.

Fine, D.L., and Arthur, L.O. Expression of Natural Antibodies against Endogenous and Horizontally Transmitted Macaque Retroviruses in Captive Primates. *Virology* 112: 49–61, 1981.

Fultz, P.N. "Simian T-lymphotropic Virus Type I." In Vol. 3, *The Retroviridae,* ed. J.A. Levy. New York: Plenum Press, 1992.

Fultz, P.N., Gordon, T.P., Anderson, D.C., and McClure, H.M. "Prevalence of Natural Infection with Simian Immunodeficiency Virus and Simian T-cell Leukemia Virus Type I in a Breeding Colony of Sooty Mangabey Monkeys." *AIDS* 4: 619–625, 1990.

Gajdusek, D.C., Gibbs, C., Jr., Epstein, L.G., Amyx, H.L., Rodgers-Johnson, P., Arthur, L.O., Gallo, R.C., Sarin, P., Montagnier, L., Mildvan, D., Mathur-Wagh, U., and Goudsmit, J. "Transmission of Human T-lymphotropic Retrovirus Infection to Chimpanzees Using Brain and Other Tissues from AIDS Patients." In *Proceedings International Congress for Infectious Diseases, Cairo, April 20–24 1985.* Rome: Luigi Pozzi, 1985.

Gallo, R.C., Salahuddin, S.Z., Popovic, M., Shearer, G.M., Kaplan, M., Haynes, B.F., Palker, T.J., Redfield, R., Oleske, J., Safai, B., White, G., Foster, P., and Markham, P.D. "Frequency Detection and Isolation of Cytopathic Retroviruses (HTLV-III) from Patients with AIDS and at Risk for AIDS. *Science* 224: 500–503, 1984.

Gallo, R.C., Sarin, P.S., Gelmann, E.P., Robert-Guroff, M., Richardson, E., Kalyanaraman, V.S., Mann, D., Sidhu, G.D., Stahl, R.E., Zolla-Pazner, S., Leibow-
itch, J., and Popovic, M. "Isolation of Human T-cell Leukemia Virus in Acquired Immune Deficiency Syndrome (AIDS)." *Science* 220: 865–867, 1983.

Gallo, R.C., Sliski, A.H., de Noronha, C.M.C., and de Noronha, F. "Origins of Human T-lymphotropic Viruses." *Nature* 320: 219, 1986.

Gallo, R.C., Sliski, A.H., and Wong-Staal, F. "Origin of Human T-cell Leukaemia-
Lymphoma Virus." *Lancet* 2(8356): 962–963, 1983.

Gao, F., Yue, L., Robertson, D.L., Hill, S.C., Hui, H., Biggar, R.J., Neequaye, A.E.,
Whelan, T.M., Ho, D.D., Shaw, G.M., Sharp, P.M., and Hahn, B.H. "Genetic Diversity of Human Immunodeficiency Virus Type 2: Evidence for Distinct Sequence Subtypes with Differences in Virus Biology." *J Virol* 11: 7433–7447, 1994.

Gardner, M.B., Endres, M., and Barry, P. "The Simian Retroviruses SIV and SRV."
In Vol. 3, *The Retroviridae*, ed. J.A. Levy. New York: Plenum Press, 1992.

Gardner, M.B., Kozak, C.A., and O'Brien, S.J. "The Lake Casitas Wild Mouse:
Evolving Genetic Resistance to Retroviral Disease." *Trends Genet* 7: 22–27, 1991.

Gartlan, J.S. "The African Coastal Rain Forest and Its Primates—Threatened Resources." In *Primate Utilization and Conservation*, ed. G. Bermant and D.G.
Lindburg. New York: Wiley, 1975.

Gautier-Hion, A., Bourlière, F., Gautier, J., and Kingdon, J., eds. *A Primate Radia-
tion: Evolutionary Biology of the African Guenons.* Cambridge: Cambridge University Press, 1988.

Gelmann, E.P., Popovic, M., Blayney, D., Masur, H., Sidhu, G., Stahl, R.E., and
Gallo, R.C. "Proviral DNA of a Retrovirus, Human T-cell Leukemia Virus, in
Two Patients with AIDS." *Science* 220: 862–865, 1983.

Gessain, A., Gallo, R.C., and Franchini, G. "Low Degree of Human T-cell
Leukemia/Lymphoma Virus Type 1 Genetic Drift in vivo as a Means of Moni-
toring Viral Transmission and Movement of Ancient Human Populations." *J Virol* 66: 2288–2295, 1992.

Gessain, A., Yanagihara, R., Franchini, G., Garruto, R.M., Jenkins, C.L.,
Ajdukiewicz, A.B., Gallo, R.C., and Gajdusek, D.C. "Highly Divergent Molecular Variants of Human T-lymphotropic Virus Type I from Isolated Populations
in Papua New Guinea and the Solomon Islands." *Proc Natl Acad Sci USA* 88:
7694–7698, 1991.

Getchell, J., Hicks, D.R., Svinivasan, A., Heath, J.L., York, D.A., Malonga, M.,
Forthal, D.N., Mann, J.M., and McCormick, J.B. "Human Immunodeficiency
Virus Isolated from a Serum Sample Collected in 1976 in Central Africa." *J In-
fect Dis* 156: 833–837, 1987.

Giddens, W.E., Jr., Tsai, C., Ochs, H.D., Knitter, G.H., and Blakley, G.A.
"Retroperitoneal Fibromatosis and Acquired Immunodeficiency Syndrome in
Macaques." *Am J Pathol* 119: 253–263, 1985.

Golovkina, T.V., Chervonsky, A., Dudley, J.P., and Ross, S.R. "Transgenic Mouse

Mammary Tumor Virus Superantigen Expression Prevents Viral Infection." *Cell* 69: 637–645, 1992.

Gonda, M.A., Boyd, A.L., Nagashima, K., and Gilden, R.V. "Pathobiology, Molecular Organization and Ultrastructure of HIV." *Arch AIDS Res* 3: 1–42, 1989.

Goudsmit, J., Back, N.K.T., and Nara, P.L. "Genomic Diversity and Antigenic Variation of HIV-1: Links between Pathogenesis, Epidemiology and Vaccine Development." *FEBS J* 5: 2427–2536, 1991.

Goudsmit, J., Debouck, C., Meloen, R.H., Smit, L., Bakker, M., Asher, D.M., Wolff, A.V., Gibbs, C., Jr., and Gajdusek, D.C. "Human Immunodeficiency Virus Type 1 Neutralization Epitope with Conserved Architecture Elicits Early Type-Specific Antibodies in Experimentally Infected Chimpanzees." *Proc Natl Acad Sci USA* 85: 4478–4482, 1988.

Goudsmit, J., Dekker, J.T., Boucher, C.A.B., Smit, L., de Ronde, A., Debouck, C., and Barin, F. "Serum Reactivity to HIV-1 Accessory Gene Products Distinguishes East African from West African HIV Strains as Infecting Agent." *AIDS Res Hum Retroviruses* 5: 457–477, 1989.

Goudsmit, J., Dekker, J., Smit, L., Kuiken, C., Geelen, J., and Perizonius, R. "Analysis of Retrovirus Sequences in c. 5300-Year-Old Egyptian Mummy DNA Obtained via PCR Amplification and Molecular Cloning." In *Biological Anthropology and the Study of Ancient Egypt*, ed. W.V. Davies and R. Walker. London: British Museum Press, 1993.

Goudsmit, J., Epstein, L.G., Paul, D.A., van der Helm, H.J., Dawson, G.J., Asher, D.M., Yanagihara, R., Wolff, A.V., Gibbs, C., Jr., and Gajdusek, D.C. "Intra-Blood-Brain Barrier Synthesis of Human Immunodeficiency Virus Antigen and Antibody in Humans and Chimpanzees." *Proc Natl Acad Sci USA* 84: 3876–3880, 1987.

Goudsmit, J., Houwers, D.J., Smit, L., and Nauta, I.M. "LAV/HTLV-III gag Gene Product p24 Shares Antigenic Determinants with Equine Infectious Anemia Virus but Not with Visna Virus or Caprine Arthritis Encephalitis Virus." *Intervirology* 26: 169–173, 1986.

Goudsmit, J., Smit, L., Krone, W.J.A., Bakker, M., van der Noordaa, J., Gibbs, C., Jr., Epstein, L.G., and Gajdusek, D.C. "IgG Response to Human Immunodeficiency Virus in Experimentally Infected Chimpanzees Mimics the IgG Response in Humans." *J Infect Dis* 155: 327–331, 1987.

Goudsmit, J., de Wolf, F., van de Wiel, B., Smit, L., Bakker, M., Albrecht–van Lent, N., and Coutinho, R.A. "Spread of Human T-cell Leukemia Virus (HTLV-I) in the Dutch Homosexual Community." *J Med Virol* 23: 115–121, 1987.

Gould, P. *The Slow Plague: A Geography of the AIDS Pandemic*. Cambridge: Blackwell, 1993.

van Griensven, G.J.P., de Vroome, E.M.M., de Wolf, F., Goudsmit, J., Roos, M., and Coutinho, R.A. "Risk Factors for Progression of Human Immunodeficiency Virus (HIV) Infection among Seroconverted Seropositive Homosexual Men."

Am J Epidemiol 132: 203–210, 1990.

van Griensven, G.J.P., de Vroome, E.M.M., Goudsmit, J., and Coutinho, R.A. "Changes in Sexual Behaviour and the Fall in Incidence of HIV Infection among Homosexual Men." *Br Med J* 298: 218–221, 1989.

van Griensven, G.J.P., Tielman, R.A., Goudsmit, J., van der Noordaa, J., de Wolf, F., de Vroome, E.M.M., and Coutinho, R.A. "Risk Factors and Prevalence of HIV Antibodies in Homosexual Men in the Netherlands." *Am J Epidemiol* 125: 1048–1057, 1987.

Grmek, M.D. *History of AIDS: Emergence and Origin of a Modern Pandemic.* Princeton, N.J.: Princeton University Press, 1990.

ten Haaft, P., Cornelissen, M., Goudsmit, J., Koornstra, W., Dubbes, R., Niphuis, H., Peeters, M., Thiriart, C., Bruck, C., and Heeney, J.L. "Virus Load in Chimpanzees Infected with Human Immunodeficiency Virus Type 1: Effect of Preexposure Vaccination." *J Gen Virol* 76: 1015–1020, 1995.

Haltenorth, T. *Säugetiere Afrikas und Madagaskars.* Munich: BLV, 1977.

Harder, T.C., Kenter, M., Appel, M.J.G., Roelke-Parker, M.E., Barrett, T., and Osterhaus, A.D.M.E. "Phylogenetic Evidence of Canine Distemper Virus in Serengeti's Lions." *Vaccine* 13: 521–523, 1995.

Hendry, R.M., Wells, M.A., Phelan, M.A., Schneider, A.L., Epstein, J.S., and Quinnan, G.V. "Antibodies to Simian Immunodeficiency Virus in African Green Monkeys in Africa in 1957–62." *Lancet* ii: 455, 1986.

Henrickson, R.V., Maul, D.H., Osborn, K.G., Sever, J.L., Madden, D.L., Ellingsworth, L.R., Anderson, J.H., Löwenstine, L.J., and Gardner, M.B. "Epidemic of Acquired Immunodeficiency in Rhesus Monkeys." *Lancet* February 19: 388–390, 1983.

Herchenröder, O., Renne, R., Loncar, D., Cobb, E.K., Murthy, K.K., Schneider, J., Mergia, A., and Luciw, P.A. "Isolation, Cloning, and Sequencing of Simian Foamy Viruses from Chimpanzees (SFVcpz): High Homology to Human Foamy Virus (HFV)." *Virology* 201: 187–199, 1994.

van den Hoek, J.A.R., Al, E.J.M., Huisman, J.G., Goudsmit, J., and Coutinho, R.A. "Low Prevalence of Human T-cell Leukaemia Virus-I and -II Infection among Drug Users in Amsterdam, the Netherlands." *J Med Virol* 34: 100–103, 1991.

van den Hoek, J.A.R., Coutinho, R.A., van Haastrecht, H.J.A., van Zadelhoff, A.W., and Goudsmit, J. "Prevalence and Risk Factors of HIV Infections among Drug Users and Drug-Using Prostitutes in Amsterdam." *AIDS* 2: 55–60, 1988.

Hogervorst, E., Jurriaans, S., de Wolf, F., van Wijk, A., Wiersma, A., Valk, M., Roos, M., van Gemen, B., Coutinho, R., Miedema, F., and Goudsmit, J. "Predictors for Non- and Slow Progression in Human Immunodeficiency Virus Type 1 Infection: Low Viral RNA Copy Numbers in Serum and Maintenance of High HIV-1 p24-specific but not V3-specific Antibody Levels." *J Infect Dis* 171: 811–821, 1995.

Hunsmann, G., Schneider, J., Schmitt, J., and Yamamoto, N. "Detection of Serum

Antibodies to Adult T-cell Leukemia Virus in Non-human Primates and in People from Africa." *Int J Cancer* 32: 329–332, 1983.

Ikeda, H., and Sugimura, H. "Fv-4 Resistance Gene: A Truncated Endogenous Murine Leukemia Virus with Ecotropic Interference Properties." *J Virol* 63: 5404–5412, 1989.

Ilyinskii, P., Daniel, M., Lerche, N.W., and Desrosiers, R. "Antibodies to Type D Retrovirus in Talapoin Monkeys." *J Gen Virol* 72: 456, 1991.

Ishida, T., Yamamoto, K., Omoto, K., Iwanaga, M., Osato, T., and Hinuma, Y. "Prevalence of a Human Retrovirus in Native Japanese: Evidence for a Possible Ancient Origin." *J Infect* 11: 153–157, 1985.

Janssens, W., Fransen, K., Peeters, M., Heyndrickx, L., Motte, J., Bedjabaga, L., Delaporte, E., Piot, P., and van der Groen, G. "Phylogenetic Analysis of a New Chimpanzee Lentivirus SIV$_{cpz\text{-}gab2}$ from a Wild-Captured Chimpanzee from Gabon." *AIDS Res Hum Retroviruses* 10: 1191–1192, 1994.

Johns, A.D., and Skorupa, J.P. "Responses of Rain-forest Primates to Habitat Disturbance: A Review." *International Journal of Primatology* 8: 157–191, 1987.

Jonckheer, T., Dab, I., van de Perre, P.H., Lepage, P.H., Dasnoy, J., and Taelman, H. "Cluster of HTLV-III/LAV Infection in an African Family." *Lancet* 1 (8425): 400–401, 1985.

Jones, J.S. "Mummified Human DNA Cloned." *Nature* 314: 576, 1985.

de Jong, J., Baan, E., Goudsmit, J., Arntzen, C.J., and Mason, H.S. "Expression of the gag Gene of HIV-1 in Potato Plants." *Vaccines*, in press.

Jurriaans, S., van Gemen, B., Weverling, G.J., van Strijp, D., Nara, P., Coutinho, R.A., Koot, M., Schuitemaker, H., and Goudsmit, J. "The Natural History of HIV-1 Infection: Virus Load and Virus Phenotype Independent Determinants of Clinical Course?" *Virology* 204: 223–233, 1994.

Kanki, P.J., Travers, K.U., M'Boup, S., Hsieh, C.C., Marlink, R.G., Gueye-Ndiaye, A., Siby, T., Thior, I., Hernandez-Avila, M., and Sankale, J.L. "Slower Heterosexual Spread of HIV-2 than HIV-1." *Lancet* 343: 943–946, 1994.

Keet, I.P.M., Krol, A., Klein, M.R., Veugelers, P., de Wit, J., Roos, M., Koot, M., Goudsmit, J., Miedema, F., and Coutinho, R.A. "Characteristics of Long-term Asymptomatic Infection with the Human Immune Deficiency Virus Type 1 with Normal and Low CD4+ Cell Counts." *J Infect Dis* 169: 1236–1243, 1994.

Keet, I.P.M., Veugelers, P.J., Koot, M., de Weerd, M.H., Roos, M.T.L., Miedema, F., de Wolf, F., Goudsmit, J., and Coutinho, R.A. "Temporal Trends of the Natural History of HIV-1 Infection Following Seroconversion between 1984 and 1993." *AIDS*, in press.

Kingsley, M. *Travels in West Africa.* London: Macmillan, 1897.

Koo, H., Gu, J., Varela-Echavarria, A., Ron, Y., and Dougherty, J.P. "Reticuloendotheliosis Type C and Primate Type D Oncoretroviruses Are Members of the Same Receptor Interference Group." *J Virol* 66: 3448–3454, 1992.

Koop, M.J. "Pneumocystis-Pneumonie: Een Studie Naar Annleiding Van Een Epidemie in Het Praematurenpaviljoen Van de St. Elisabethkliniek te Heerlen." Thesis, Heerlen: Winants, 1964.

Koralnik, I.J., Boeri, E., Saxinger, W.C., Monico, A.L., Fullen, J., Gessain, A., Guo, H., Gallo, R.C., Markham, P., Kalyanaraman, V., Hirsch, V., Allan, J., Murthy, K., Alford, P., Slattery, J.P., O'Brien, S.J., and Franchini, G. "Phylogenetic Associations of Human and Simian T-cell Leukemia/Lymphotropic Virus Type I Strains: Evidence for Interspecies Transmission." *J Virol* 68: 2693–2707, 1994.

Kozak, C.A., Gromet, N.J., Ikeda, H., and Buckler, C.E. "A Unique Sequence Related to the Ecotropic Murine Leukemia Virus Is Associated with the Fv-4 Resistance Gene." *Proc Natl Acad Sci USA* 81: 834–837, 1984.

Kuiken, C., Lukashov, V.V., Cornelissen, M., and Goudsmit, J. "HIV Variability and Its Implications for Epidemiology, Natural History and Pathogenesis." In *Global Challenge of AIDS—Ten Years of HIV/AIDS Research* (proceedings of the 10th International Conference on AIDS and STD, Yokohama, August 7–12 1994), ed. Y. Shiokawa and T. Kitamura. Tokyo: Kodansha Scientific, 1995.

Kuiken, C.L., and Goudsmit, J. "Silent Mutation Pattern in V3 Sequences Distinguishes Virus According to Risk Group in Europe." *AIDS Res Hum Retroviruses* 10: 319–320, 1994.

Kuiken, C.L., van Griensven, G.J.P., de Vroome, E.M.M., and Coutinho, R.A. "Risk Factors and Changes in Sexual Behavior in Male Homosexuals Who Seroconverted for Human Immunodeficiency Virus Antibodies." *Am J Epidemiol* 132: 523–530, 1990.

Kuiken, C.L., Nieselt-Struwe, K., Weiller, G.F., and Goudsmit, J. "Quasispecies Behavior of HIV-1: A Sample Analysis of Sequence Data." In *Methods in Molecular Genetics*, vol. 4: *Molecular Virology*, ed. K.W. Adolph. Orlando: Academic Press, 1994.

Kuiken, C.L., Zwart, G., Baan, E., Coutinho, R.A., van den Hoek, J.A.R., and Goudsmit, J. "Increasing Antigenic and Genetic Diversity of the V3 Variable Domain of the Human Immunodeficiency Virus Envelope Protein in the Course of the AIDS Epidemic." *Proc Natl Acad Sci USA* 90: 9061–9065, 1993.

van der Kuyl, A.C., Dekker, J., Attia, M.A.M., Iskander, N., Perizonius, W.R.K., and Goudsmit, J. "DNA from Ancient Egyptian Monkey Bones." *Ancient DNA Newsletter* 2: 19–21, 1994.

van der Kuyl, A.C., Dekker, J., Clutton-Brock, J., Perizonius, W.R.K., and Goudsmit, J. "Sequence Analysis of Mitochondrial DNA Fragments from Mummified Egyptian Monkey Tissue." *Ancient DNA Newsletter* 1: 17–18, 1992.

van der Kuyl, A.C., Dekker, J., and Goudsmit, J. "Full-Length Proviruses of Baboon Endogenous Virus (BaEV) and Dispersed BaEV Reverse Transcriptase Retroelements in the Genome of Baboon Species." *J Virol* 69: 5917–5924, 1995a.

van der Kuyl, A.C., Dekker, J., and Goudsmit, J. "Distribution of Baboon Endogenous Virus among Species of African Monkeys Suggests Multiple Ancient Cross-Species Transmissions in Shared Habitats." *J Virol* 69: 7877–7887, 1995b.

van der Kuyl, A.C., Kuiken, C.L., Dekker, J.T., and Goudsmit, J. "Phylogeny of African Monkeys Based upon Mitochondrial 12S rRNA Sequences." *J Mol Evol* 40: 173–180, 1995.

van der Kuyl, A.C., Kuiken, C.L., Dekker, J.T., Perizonius, W.R.K., and Goudsmit, J. "Nuclear Counterparts of the Cytoplasmic Mitochondrial 12S rRNA Gene: A Problem of Ancient DNA and Molecular Phylogenies." *J Mol Evol* 40: 657, 1995.

Lange, J.M.A., Teeuwsen, V.J.P., Boucher, C.A.B., Vahlne, A., Barin, F., Tjong-A-Hung, S., Dekker, J., Parkhede, U., de Wolf, F., and Goudsmit, J. Antigenic Variation of the Dominant gp41 Epitope in Africa." *AIDS* 7: 461–466, 1993.

Lee, P.C., Thornback, J., and Bennett, E.L. *Threatened Primates of Africa*. Gland: International Union for Conservation of Nature and Natural Resources, 1988.

Lerche, N.W., Henrickson, R.V., Maul, D.H., and Gardner, M.B. "Epidemiologic Aspects of an Outbreak of Acquired Immunodeficiency in Rhesus Monkeys (*Macaca mulatta*)." *Lab Anim Sci* 34: 146–150, 1984.

Lerche, N.W., Marx, P.A., Osborn, K.G., Maul, D.H., Löwenstine, L.J., Bleviss, M.L., Moody, P., Henrickson, R.V., and Gardner, M.B. "Natural History of Endemic Type D Retrovirus Infection and Acquired Immune Deficiency Syndrome in Group-Housed Rhesus Monkeys." *J Natl Cancer Inst* 79: 847–854, 1987.

Lerche, N.W., Osborn, K.G., Marx, P.A., Prahalada, S., Maul, D.H., Löwenstine, L.J., Munn, R.J., Bryant, M.L., Henrickson, R.V., Arthur, L.O., Gilden, R.V., Barker, C.S., Hunter, E., and Gardner, M.B. "Inapparent Carriers of Simian Acquired Immune Deficiency Syndrome Type D Retrovirus and Disease Transmission with Saliva." *J Natl Cancer Inst* 77: 489–495, 1986.

Lerner, D.L., Wagaman, P.C., Phillips, T.R., Prospero-Garcia, O., Henriksen, S.J., Fox, H.S., Bloom, F.E., and Elder, J.H. "Increased Mutation Frequency of Feline Immunodeficiency Virus Lacking Functional Deoxyuridine-Triphosphatase." *Proc Natl Acad Sci USA* 92: 7480–7484, 1995.

Levy, J.A., Pan, L., Beth-Giraldo, E., Kaminsky, L.S., Henle, G., Henle, W., and Giraldo, G. "Absence of Antibodies to the Human Immunodeficiency Virus in Sera from Africa Prior to 1975." *Proc Natl Acad Sci USA* 83: 7935–7937, 1986.

Lewis, D. *Jan Compagnie in the Straits of Malacca 1641–1795*. Athens, OH: Ohio University Center for International Studies, 1995.

de Leys, R., Vanderborght, B., van den Haesevelde, M., Heyndrickx, L., van Geel, A., Wauters, C., Bernaerts, R., Saman, E., Nijs, P., Willems, B., Taelman, H., van der Groen, G., Piot, P., Tersmette, M., Huisman, J.G., and van Heuverswijn, H. "Isolation and Partial Characterization of an Unusual Human Immunodeficiency Retrovirus from Two Persons of West-Central African Origin." *J Virol* 64: 1207–1216, 1990.

van Lier, R.A.J. Samenleving in een Grensgebied: Een sociaal-historische studie van de maatschappij in Suriname. Gravenhage: Nijhoff, 1949.

van der Loo, E.M., van Muijen, G.N.P., van Vloten, W.A., Beens, W., Scheffer, E., and Meijer, C.J.L.M. "C-type Virus-like Particles Specifically Localized in Langerhans' Cells and Related Cells of Skin and Lymph Nodes of Patients with Mycosis Fungoides and Sézary's Syndrome." *Virchows Arch B Cell Pathol* 31: 193–203, 1979.

Lukashov, V.V., Cornelissen, M.T.E., Goudsmit, J., Papuashvili, M.N., Rytik, P.G., Khaitov, R.M., Karamov, E.V., and de Wolf, F. "Simultaneous Introduction of Distinct HIV-1 Subtypes into Different Risk Groups in Russia, Byelorussia and Lithuania." *AIDS* 9: 435–439, 1995.

Lukashov, V.V., and Goudsmit, J. "Increasing Genotypic and Phenotypic Selection from the Original Genomic RNA Population of HIV-1 Strains LAI and MN (NM) by Peripheral Blood Mononuclear Cell Culture, B-cell-Line Propagation and T-cell-Line Adaption." *AIDS* 9: 1307–1311, 1995.

———. "Evolution of the Human Immunodeficiency Virus Type 1 Subtype-Specific V3 Domain Is Confined to a Sequence with a Fixed Distance to the Subtype Consensus." Journal of Virology 71: 6332–6338, 1997.

Lukashov, V.V., Kuiken, C., and Goudsmit, J. "Intrahost Human Immunodeficiency Virus Type 1 Evolution Is Related to Length of the Immunocompetent Period." *J Virol* 69: 6911–6916, 1995.

Lukashov, V.V., Kuiken, C.L., Vlahov, D., Coutinho, R.A., and Goudsmit, J. "Evidence for HIV-1 Strains of US IV Drug Users as Founders of AIDS Epidemic among IV Drug Users in Northern Europe." *AIDS Res Hum Retroviruses* 12: 1179–1183.

Luo, C., Tian, C.Q., Hu, D.J., and Kai, M. "HIV-1 Subtype C in China." *Lancet* 345: 1051–1052, 1995.

Lusso, P., di Marzo Veronese, F., Ensoli, B., Franchini, G., Jemma, C., DeRocco, S.E., Kalyanaraman, V.S., and Gallo, R.C. "Expanded HIV-1 Cellular Tropism by Phenotypic Mixing with Murine Endogenous Retroviruses." *Science* 247: 848–852, 1990.

Mansfield, K.G., Lerche, N.W., Gardner, M.B., and Lackner, A.A. "Origins of Simian Immunodeficiency Virus Infection in Macaques at the New England Regional Primate Research Center." *J Med Primatol* 24: 116–122, 1995.

Marlink, R., Kanki, P., Thior, I., Travers, K., Eisen, G., Siby, T., Traore, I., Hsieh, C., Dia, M.C., Gueye, E, Hellinger, J., Guèye-Ndiaye, A., Sankalé, J., Ndoye, I., M'Boup, S., and Essex, M. "Reduced Rate of Disease Development after HIV-2 Infection as Compared to HIV-1." *Science* 265: 1587–1590, 1996.

Marx, P.A., Bryant, M.L., Osborn, K.G., Maul, D.H., Lerche, N.W., Löwenstine, L.J., Kluge, J.D., Zaiss, C.P., Henrickson, R.V., Shiigi, S.M., Wilson, B.J., Malley, A., Olson, L.C., McNulty, W.P., Arthur, L.O., Gilden, R.V., Barker, C.S., Hunter, E., Munn, R.J., Heidecker, G., and Gardner, M.B. "Isolation of a New Serotype of Simian Acquired Immune Deficiency Syndrome Type D Retrovirus from Celebes Black Macaques (*Macaca nigra*) with Immune Deficiency and Retroperitoneal Fibromatosis." *J Virol* 56: 571–578, 1985.

Marx, P.A., Maul, D.H., Osborn, K.G., Lerche, N.W., Moody, P., Löwenstine, L.J., Henrickson, R.V., Arthur, L.O., Gilden, R.V., Gravell, M., London, W.T., Sever, J.L., Levy, J.A., Munn, R.J., and Gardner, M.B. "Simian AIDS: Isolation of a Type D Retrovirus and Transmission of the Disease." *Science* 223: 1085, 1984.

McClure, M.A., Johnson, M.S., Feng, D.F., and Doolittle, R.F. "Sequence Comparisons of Retroviral Proteins: Relative Rates of Change and General Phylogeny." *Proc Natl Acad Sci USA* 85: 2469–2473, 1988.

McEvedy, C. *The Penguin Atlas of African History.* London: Penguin, 1980.

van der Meeberg, P.C., Kooiman, R.C., Buisman, N.J.F., Goudsmit, J., Lange, J.M.A., and Bannenberg, A.F.I. "The Prevalence of Human Immunodeficiency Virus among Pregnant Women Attending a Hospital in the Moungo District, Cameroon." *Trop Geogr Med* 41: 45–48, 1989.

Mergia, A., and Luciw, P.A. "Replication and Regulation of Primate Foamy Viruses." *Virology* 184: 475–482, 1991.

Mergia, A., Shaw, K.E.S., Lackner, J.E., and Luciw, P.A. "Relationship of the env Genes and the Endonuclease Domain of the pol Genes of Simian Foamy Virus Type 1 and Human Foamy Virus." *J Virol* 64: 406–410, 1990.

Miedema, F., Chantal Petit, A.J., Terpstra, F.G., Eeftinck Schattenkerk, J.K.M., de Wolf, F., Al, B.J.M., Roos, M.T.L., Lange, J.M.A., Danner, S.A., Goudsmit, J., and Schellekens, P.T.H. "Immunological Abnormalities in Human Immunodeficiency Virus (HIV)-Infected Asymptomatic Homosexual Men." *J Clin Invest* 82: 1908–1914, 1988.

Mientjes, G.H.C., van Ameijden, E.J.C., Miedema, F., van den Hoek, J.A.R., Goudsmit, J., and Coutinho, R.A. "Progression of HIV Infection among Injecting Drug Users: Indications for a Lower Rate of Progression among Those Who Have Frequently Borrowed Injecting Equipment." *AIDS* 7: 1363–1370, 1993.

Morell, V. "Mystery Ailment Strikes Serengeti Lions." *Science* 264: 1404, 1994.

———. "Serengeti's Big Cats Going to the Dogs." *Science* 264: 1664, 1994.

Morse, S.S., ed. *The Evolutionary Biology of Viruses.* New York: Raven Press, 1994.

Mulder-Kampinga, G.A., Simonon, A., Kuiken, C., Dekker, J., Scherpbier, H.J., van de Perre, P., Boer, K., and Goudsmit, J. "Similarity in env and gag Genes between Genomic RNA of Human Immunodeficiency Virus Type 1 (HIV-1) from Mother and Infant Is Unrelated to Time of HIV-1 RNA Positivity in the Child." *J Virol* 69: 2285–2296, 1995.

Myers, G. "HIV: Between Past and Future." *AIDS Res Hum Retroviruses* 11: 1317–1324, 1994.

Nahmias, A.J., Weiss, J., Yao, X., Lee, F., Kodsi, R., Schanfield, M., Matthews, T., Bolognesi, D., Durack, D., Motulsky, A., Kanki, P., and Essex, M. "Evidence for Human Infection with an HTLV III/LAV-like Virus in Central Africa, 1959." *Lancet* 1(8492): 1279–1280, 1986.

Napier, J.R., and Napier, P.H. *The Natural History of the Primates.* Cambridge: Cambridge University Press, 1985.

Nerurkar, V.R., Song, K., Bastian, I.V., Garin, B., Franchini, G., and Yanagihara, R. "Genotyping of Human T Cell Lymphotropic Virus Type I Using Australo-Melanesian Topotype-Specific Oligonucleotide Primer-based Polymerase Chain Reaction: Insights into Viral Evolution and Dissemination." *J Infect Dis* 170: 1353–1360, 1994.

Nerurkar, V.R., Song, K., Melland, R.R., and Yanagihara, R. "Genetic and Phylogenetic Analyses of Human T-cell Lymphotropic Virus Type I Variants from Melanesians with and without Spastic Myelopathy." *Mol Neurobiol* 8: 155–173, 1994.

Nkengasong, J., Janssens, W., Heyndrickx, L., Fransen, K., Ndumbe, P.M., Motte, J., Leonaers, A., Ngolle, M., Ayuk, J., Piot, P., and van der Groen, G. "Genotypic Subtypes of HIV-1 in Cameroon." *AIDS* 8: 1405–1412, 1994.

Olmsted, R.A., Langley, R., Roelke, M.E., Goeken, R.M., Adger-Johnson, D., Goff, J.P., Albert, J., Packer, C., Laurenson, M.K., Caro, T.M., Scheepers, L., Wildt, D.E., Bush, M., Martensson, J.S., and O'Brien, S.J. "Worldwide Prevalence of Lentivirus Infection in Wild Feline Species: Epidemiologic and Phylogenetic Aspects." *J Virol* 66: 6008–6018, 1992.

Pääbo, S. "Molecular Cloning of Ancient Egyptian Mummy DNA." *Nature* 314: 644–645, 1985.

———. "Ancient DNA: Extraction, Characterization, Molecular Cloning, and Enzymatic Amplification." *Proc Natl Acad Sci USA* 86: 1939–1943, 1989.

Pääbo, S., Higuchi, R.G., and Wilson, A.C. "Ancient DNA and the Polymerase Chain Reaction." *J Biol Chem* 264: 9709–9712, 1989.

Pääbo, S., Irwin, D.M., and Wilson, A.C. "DNA Damage Promotes Jumping between Templates during Enzymatic Amplification." *J Biol Chem* 265: 4718–4721, 1990.

Pakenham, T. *The Scramble for Africa: White Man's Conquest of the Dark Continent from 1876 to 1912.* New York: Avon, 1992.

Pan, L. *Sons of the Yellow Emperor: A History of the Chinese Diaspora.* New York: Kodansha International, 1994.

Peeters, M., Fransen, K., Delaporte, E., van den Haesevelde, M., Gershy-Damet, G.M., Kestens, L., van der Groen, G., and Piot, P. "Isolation and Characterization of a New Chimpanzee Lentivirus (Simian Immunodeficiency Virus Isolate cpz-ant) from a Wild-Captured Chimpanzee." *AIDS* 6: 447–451, 1992.

Perizonius, R., Attia, M., Smith, H., and Goudsmit, J. "Monkey Mummies and North Saqqara." *Egyptian Archaeology* 3: 31–33, 1993.

Picard, F.J., Coulthart, M.B., Oger, J., King, E.E., Kim, S., Arp, J., Rice, G.P.A., and Dekaban, GA. "Human T-lymphotropic Virus Type I in Coastal Natives of British Columbia: Phylogenetic Affinities and Possible Origins." *J Virol* 69: 7248–7256, 1995.

van de Pitte, J., Verwilghen, R., and Zachee, P. "AIDS and Cryptococcosis (Zaire, 1977)." *Lancet* 1 (8330): 925–926, 1983.

Popovic, M., Sarngadharan, M.G., Read, E., and Gallo, R.C. "Detection, Isolation, and Continuous Production of Cytopathic Retroviruses (HTLV-III) from Patients with AIDS and Pre-AIDS." *Science* 224: 497–500, 1984.

Quaegobeur, J. "Les Singes et la Représentation de Leurs Pieds en Égypte Ancienne." *Acta Archaeologica Lovaniensia* 32: 3–28, 1993.

Querat, G., Audoly, G., Sonigo, P., and Vigne, R. "Nucleotide Sequence Analysis of SA-OMVV, a Visna-Related Ovine Lentivirus: Phylogenetic History of Lentiviruses." *Virology* 175: 434–447, 1990.

Ridley, M. *The Red Queen: Sex and the Evolution of Human Nature.* London: Penguin, 1993.

Robertson, D.L., Sharp, P.M., McCutchan, F.E., and Hahn, B.H. "Recombination in HIV-1." *Nature* 374: 124–126, 1995.

Robinson, H.L., Astrin, S.M., Senior, A.M., and Salazar, F.H. "Host Susceptibility to Endogenous Viruses: Defective Glycoprotein-Expressing Proviruses Interfere with Infections." *J Virol* 40: 745–751, 1981.

Rodhain, J., and van den Berghe, L. "Contribution a L'étude des Plasmodiums des Singes Africains." *Ann Soc Belg Med Trop* 36: 521–531, 1936.

Rodhain, J., and Dellaert, R. "L'Infection à *Plasmodium schwetzi* chez l'homme." *Ann Soc Belg Med Trop* 46:757–771, 1955.

Rubin, E., and Zak, F.G. "*Pneumocystis carinii* Pneumonia in the Adult." *N Engl J Med* 262: 1315–1317, 1960.

Sabater, J., and Groves, C. "The Importance of Higher Primates in the Diet of the Fang of Rio Muni." *Man* 7: 239–243, 1972.

Saksena, N.K., Herve, V., Durand, J.P., Leguenno, B., Diop, O.M., Digoute, J.P., Mathiot, C., Muller, M.C., Love, J.L., Dube, S., Sherman, M.P., Benz, P.M., Erensoy, S., Galat-Luong, A., Galat, G., Paul, B., Dube, D.K., Barré-Sinoussi, F., and Poiesz, B.J. "Seroepidemiologic, Molecular and Phylogenetic Analyses of Simian T-cell Leukemia Viruses (STLV-1) from Various Naturally Infected Monkey Species from Central and Western Africa." *Virology* 198: 297–310, 1994.

Samuelson, L.C., Wiebauer, K., Snow, C.M., and Meisler, M.H. "Retroviral and Pseudogene Insertion Sites Reveal the Lineage of Human Salivary and Pancreatic Amylase Genes from a Single Gene during Primate Evolution." *Mol Cell Biol* 10: 2513–2520, 1990.

Sayer, J.A., Harcourt, C.S., and Collins, N.M., eds. *The Conservation Atlas of Tropical Forests—Africa.* New York: Simon and Schuster, 1992.

Schweizer, M., and Neumann-Maefelin, D. "Phylogenetic Analysis of Primate Foamy Viruses by Comparison of pol Sequences." *Virology* 207: 577–582, 1995.

Seifarth, W., Skladny, H., Krieg-Schneider, F., Reichert, A., Hehlmann, R., and Leib-Mösch, C. "Retrovirus-like Particles Released from the Human Breast Cancer Cell Line T47-D Display Type B– and C–Related Endogenous Retroviral Sequences." *J Virol* 69: 6408–6416, 1995.

de Sélincourt, A., and Burn, A.R., eds. *Herodotus: The Histories*. London: Penguin, 1972.

Serwadda, D., Sewankambo, N.K., Carswell, J.W., Bayley, A.C., Tedder, R.S., Weiss, R.A., Mugerwa, R.D., Lwegaba, A., Kirya, G.B., Downing, R.G., Clayden, S.A., and Dalgleish, A.G. "Slim Disease: A New Disease in Uganda and Its Association with HTLV-III Infection." *Lancet* 2 (8460): 849–852, 1985.

Sharp, P.M., Robertson, D.L., and Hahn, B.H. "Cross-Species Transmission and Recombination of AIDS Viruses." *Philos Trans R Soc Lond Biol* 349: 41–47, 1995.

Sherman, M.P., Saksena, N.K., Dube, D.K., Yanagihara, R., and Poiesz, B.J. "Evolutionary Insight on the Origin of Human T-cell Lymphoma/Leukemia Virus Type 1 (HTLV-I) Derived from Sequence Analysis of a New HTLV-I Variant from Papua New Guinea." *J Virol* 66: 2556–2563, 1992.

Simon, F., Matheron, S., Tamalet, C., Loussert-Ajaka, I., Bartczak, S., Pépin, J.M., Dhiver, C., Gamba, E., Elbim, C., Gastaut, J.A., Saimot, A.G., and Brun-Vézinet, F. "Cellular and Plasma Viral Load in Patients Infected with HIV-2." *AIDS* 7: 1411–1417, 1993.

Sinclair, A.R.E., and Arcese, P., eds. *Serengeti II: Dynamic, Management and Conservation of an Ecosystem*. Chicago: University of Chicago Press, 1995.

Smith, H.S. "Walter Bryan Emery." *Journal of Egyptian Archaeology* 57: 190–201, 1971.

———. *A Visit to Ancient Egypt: Life at Memphis and Saqqara (c. 500–30 BC)*. Warminster: Aris and Phillips, 1974.

Smuts, B.B., Cheney, D.L., Seyfarth, R.M., Srangham, R.W., and Struksaker, T.T., eds. *Primate Societies*. Chicago: University of Chicago Press, 1987.

Sommerfelt, M.A., and Weiss, R.A. "Receptor Interference Groups of 20 Retroviruses Plating on Human Cells." *Virology* 176: 58–69, 1990.

Song, K., Nerurkar, V.R., Pereira-Cortez, A.J., Yamamoto, M., Taguchi, H., Miyoshi, I., and Yanagihara, R. "Sequence and Phylogenetic Analyses of Human T Cell Lymphotropic Virus Type I from a Brazilian Woman with Adult T Cell Leukemia: Comparison with Virus Strains from South America and the Caribbean Basin." *Am J Trop Med Hyg* 52: 101–108, 1995.

Stellingwerff, J. *De Diepe Wateren van Nagasaki*. Franeker: Uitgeverij T. Wever b.v. 1983.

Stoye, J.P., and Coffin, J.M. "The Four Classes of Endogenous Murine Leukemia Virus: Structural Relationships and Potential for Recombination." *J Virol* 61: 2659–2669, 1987.

Stromberg, K., Benveniste, R.E., Arthur, L.O., Rabin, H., Giddens, W.E., Jr., Ochs, H.D., Morton, W.R., and Tsai, C. "Characterization of Exogenous Type D Retrovirus from a Fibroma of a Macaque with Simian AIDS and Fibromatosis." *Science* 224: 289–292, 1984.

Temin, H.M. "Sex and Recombination in Retroviruses." *Trends Genet* 7: 71–74, 1991.

Ting, C., Rosenberg, M.P., Snow, C.M., Samuelson, L., and Meisler, M.H. "Endogenous Retroviral Sequences Are Required for Tissue-Specific Expression of a Human Salivary Amylase Gene." *Genes Dev* 8: 1457–1465, 1992.

Todaro, G.J., Benveniste, R.E., Sherr, C.J., Schlom, J., Schidlovsky, G., and Stephenson, J.R. "Isolation and Characterization of a New Type D Retrovirus from the Asian Primate, *Presbytis obscurus* (Spectacled Langur)." *Virology* 84: 189–194, 1978.

Todaro, G.J., Sherr, C.J., and Benveniste, R.E. "Baboons and Their Close Relatives Are Unusual among Primates in Their Ability to Release Nondefective Endogenous Type C Viruses." *Virology* 72: 278–282, 1976.

Traina-Dorge, V., Blanchard, J., Martin, L., and Murphey-Corb, M. "Immunodeficiency and Lymphoproliferative Disease in an African Green Monkey Dually Infected with SIV and STLV-I." *AIDS Res Hum Retroviruses* 8: 97–100, 1992.

Travers, K., M'Boup, S., Marlink, R., Guèye-Ndiaye, A., Siby, T., Thior, I., Traore, I., Dieng-Sarr, A., Sankalé, J., Mullins, C., Ndoye, I., Hsieh, C., Essex, M., and Kanki, P. "Natural Protection against HIV-1 Infection Provided by HIV-2." *Science* 268: 1612–1615, 1995.

Tsujimoto, H., Hasegawa, A., Maki, N., Fukasawa, M., Miura, T., Speidel, S., Cooper, R.W., Moriyama, E.N., Gojobori, T., and Hayami, M. "Sequence of a Novel Simian Immunodeficiency Virus from a Wild-Caught African Mandrill." *Nature* 341: 539–541, 1989.

Turner, C.G., II. "Teeth and Prehistory in Asia." *Scientific American* 260: 88–91, 1989.

Veugelers, P.J., Page, K.A., Tindall, B., Schechter, M.T., Moss, A.R., Winkelstein, W.W., Jr., Cooper, D.A., Craib, K.J.P., Charlebois, E., Coutinho, R.A., and van Griensven, G.J.P. "Determinants of HIV Disease Progression among Homosexual Men Registered in the Tricontinental Seroconverter Study." *Am J Epidemiol* 140: 747–757, 1994.

Williams, G., Stretton, T.B., and Leonard, J.C. "Cytomegalic Inclusion Disease and *Pneumocystis carinii* Infection in an Adult." *Lancet* October 29: 951–955, 1960.

de Wolf, F., Hogervorst, E., Goudsmit, J., Fenyö, E.M., Rübsamen-Waigmann, H., Holmes, H., Galvao-Castro, B., Karita, E., Wasi, C., Sempala, S.D.K., Baan, E., Zorgdrager, F., Lukashov, V., Osmanov, S., Kuiken, C., Cornelissen, M., and WHO Network on HIV-1 Isolation and Characterization. "Syncytium Inducing (SI) and Non-Syncytium Inducing (NSI) Capacity of Human Immunodeficiency Virus Type 1 (HIV-1) Subtypes Other Than B: Phenotypic and Genotypic Characteristics." *AIDS Res Hum Retroviruses* 10: 1387–1400, 1994.

de Wolf, F., Meloen, R.H., Bakker, M., Barin, F., and Goudsmit, J. "Characterization of Human Antibody-Binding Sites on the External Envelope of Human Immunodeficiency Virus Type 2." *J Gen Virol* 72: 1261–1267, 1991.

Wolfs, T.F.W., de Jong, J.J., van den Berg, H., Tijnagel, J.M.G.H., Krone, W.J.A., and Goudsmit, J. "Evolution of Sequences Encoding the Principal Neutralization Epitope of HIV-1 Is Host-Dependent, Rapid and Continuous." *Proc Natl Acad Sci USA* 87: 9938–9942, 1990.

Wolfs, T.F.W., Zwart, G., Bakker, M., and Goudsmit, J. "HIV-1 Genomic RNA Diversification Following Sexual and Parental Virus Transmission." *Virology* 189: 103–110, 1992.

Yamashita, M., Kitze, B., Miura, T., Weber, T., Fujiyoshi, T., Takehisa, J., Chen, J.L., Sonoda, S., and Hayami, M. "The Phylogenetic Relationship of HTLV Type I from Non-Mashhadi Iranians to That from Mashhadi Jews." *AIDS Res Hum Retroviruses* 11: 1533–1535, 1995.

Zhu, T.F., and Ho, D.D. "Was HIV Present in 1959?" *Nature* 374: 503–504, 1995.

Zwart, G., de Jong, J., Wolfs, T., van der Hoek, L., Smit, L., de Ronde, A., Tersmette, M., Nara, P., and Goudsmit, J. "Predominance of HIV-1 Serotype Distinct from LAV-1/HTLV-IIIB." *Lancet* 335: 474, 1990.

Zwart, G., Wolfs, T.F.W., Bookelman, R., Hartman, S., Bakker, M., Boucher, C.A.B., Kuiken, C., and Goudsmit, J. "Greater Diversity of the HIV-1 V3 Neutralization Domain in Tanzania Compared with the Netherlands: Serological and Genetic Analysis." *AIDS* 7: 467–474, 1993.

Index

12.26